Computed Tomography of the Musculoskeletal System

Contemporary Issues in Computed Tomography
Volume 8

SERIES EDITOR

Elliot K. Fishman, M.D.
Associate Professor
The Russell H. Morgan Department of Radiology and Radiological Science
Director, Division of Computed Body Tomography
The Johns Hopkins Medical Institutions
Baltimore, Maryland

Volumes Already Published

Forthcoming Volumes in the Series

Computed Tomography of the Musculoskeletal System

Edited by

William W. Scott, Jr., M.D.

Associate Professor
The Russell H. Morgan Department of Radiology and Radiological Science
Director of Musculoskeletal Imaging
Director of Medical Student Education in Radiology
The Johns Hopkins Medical Institutions
Baltimore, Maryland

Donna Magid, M.D.

Assistant Professor
The Russell H. Morgan Department of Radiology and Radiological Science
Division of Musculoskeletal Imaging
Assistant Professor
Orthopaedic Surgery
The Johns Hopkins Medical Institutions
Baltimore, Maryland

Elliot K. Fishman, M.D.

Associate Professor
The Russell H. Morgan Department of Radiology and Radiological Science
Director, Division of Computed Body Tomography
The Johns Hopkins Medical Institutions
Baltimore, Maryland

CHURCHILL LIVINGSTONE
NEW YORK, EDINBURGH, LONDON, MELBOURNE
1987

Library of Congress Cataloging-in-Publication Data

Computed tomography of the musculoskeletal system.
  Contemporary issues in computed tomography; 8)
  Bibliography: p.
  Includes index.
  1. Musculoskeletal system—Diseases—Diagnosis.
2. Tomography. I. Scott, William W. (William
Wallace), date. II. Magid, Donna.
III. Fishman, Elliot K. IV. Series. [DNLM:
1. Musculoskeletal System—radiography. 2. Tomography,
X-Ray Computed. W1 C0769MQK v.8 / WE 141 C7385]
RC925.7.C66 1987   616.7'07'572   86–21590
ISBN 0 443-08497-1

© **Churchill Livingstone Inc. 1987**

Distributed in the United Kingdom by Churchill Livingstone, Robert
Stevenson House, 1–3 Baxter's Place, Leith Walk, Edinburgh EH1 3AF,
and by associated companies, branches, and representatives
throughout the world.

Accurate indications, adverse reactions, and dosage schedules for drugs
are provided in this book, but it is possible that they may change.
The reader is urged to review the package information data of the
manufacturers of the medications mentioned.

Acquisitions Editor: *Kim Loretucci*
Copy Editor: *Patricia Rind*
Production Designer: *Michiko Davis*
Production Supervisor: *Jocelyn Eckstein*

Printed in the United States of America

First published in 1987

To our children—

Whitney Skyler
and
Kevin, Sarah, and Mark

Contributors

Rudolph Almaraz, M.D.
Assistant Professor of Surgery and Oncology, The Johns Hopkins University School of Medicine, Baltimore, Maryland

Thomas J. Beck, Sc.M.
Instructor in Radiology, The Russell H. Morgan Department of Radiology and Radiological Science, The Johns Hopkins University School of Medicine, Baltimore, Maryland

Charles Diana, M.D.
Fellow in Diagnostic Radiology, The Russell H. Morgan Department of Radiology and Radiological Science, Johns Hopkins Hospital, Baltimore, Maryland

Bob Drebin, M.D.
Research and Development Scientist, PIXAR INC., San Rafael, California

Faith Farley, M.D.
Fellow in Diagnostic Radiology, The Russell H. Morgan Department of Radiology and Radiological Science, The Johns Hopkins Hospital, Baltimore, Maryland

Edward Farmlett, M.D.
Fellow in Diagnostic Radiology, The Russell H. Morgan Department of Radiology and Radiological Science, The Johns Hopkins Hospital, Baltimore, Maryland

Elliot K. Fishman, M.D.
Associate Professor, The Russell H. Morgan Department of Radiology and Radiological Science; Director, Division of Computed Body Tomography, The Johns Hopkins Medical Institutions, Baltimore, Maryland

Steven E. Harms, M.D.
Director of Magnetic Resonance, Department of Medical Imaging, Baylor University Medical Center, Dallas, Texas

Janet Kuhlman, M.D.
Fellow in Diagnostic Radiology, The Russell H. Morgan Department of Radiology and Radiological Science, The Johns Hopkins Hospital, Baltimore, Maryland

Alma Lynch-Nyhan, M.D.
Fellow in Diagnostic Radiology, The Russell H. Morgan Department of Radiology and Radiological Science, The Johns Hopkins Hospital, Baltimore, Maryland

Donna Magid, M.D.
Assistant Professor, The Russell H. Morgan Department of Radiology and Radiological Science, Division of Musculoskeletal Imaging; Assistant Professor of Orthopaedic Surgery, The Johns Hopkins Medical Institutions, Baltimore, Maryland

Richard P. Moser, Jr., L.T.C., M.C., U.S.A.
Associate Professor of Clinical Radiology and Nuclear Medicine, Uniformed Services University of the Health Sciences, Bethesda, Maryland; Chairman and Registrar, Department of Radiologic Pathology, Armed Forces Institute of Pathology, Washington, D.C.

Gopala U. Rao, Sc.D.
Associate Professor, The Russell H. Morgan Department of Radiology and Radiological Science, The Johns Hopkins University School of Medicine, Baltimore, Maryland

Charles S. Resnik, M.D.
Associate Professor of Radiology, University of Maryland Hospital, Baltimore, Maryland

Douglas D. Robertson, M.D.
Assistant Professor, Department of Orthopedic Surgery, Harvard Medical School, Boston, Massachusetts

William W. Scott, Jr., M.D.
Associate Professor, The Russell H. Morgan Department of Radiology and Radiological Science; Director of Musculoskeletal Imaging and Director of Medical Student Education in Radiology, The Johns Hopkins Medical Institutions, Baltimore, Maryland

David M. Yousem, M.D.
Chief Resident in Radiology, The Russell H. Morgan Department of Radiology and Radiological Science, Division of Musculoskeletal Imaging, The Johns Hopkins Hospital, Baltimore, Maryland

Eva S. Zinreich, M.D.
Assistant Professor of Oncology and Radiology, The Johns Hopkins University School of Medicine, Baltimore, Maryland

Preface

Computed tomography (CT) has revolutionized the diagnostic evaluation of musculoskeletal pathology. In the future, magnetic resonance imaging (MRI) will almost certainly modify the workup of skeletal problems, but CT will long remain one of the major elements of the diagnostic imaging evaluation. The relative high cost and limited availability of MRI, the current ubiquity of CT, and the increasing concern with medical costs insure the importance of CT in this area for several years to come.

In keeping with the general intention of this series, we have assembled a text focused on a specific application of computed tomography—in this case, musculoskeletal imaging. This text encompasses a review of current techniques, including arthrotomography and multiplanar reformatting, and a review of the capabilities still evolving, including dual energy assessment of osteoporosis, three-dimensional image generation, and three-dimensional analysis for biomechanically optimal orthopedic prosthetic design. Representative cases are chosen throughout to illustrate and to reinforce the basic principles of the text.

We wish to thank Dr. Stanley S. Siegelman for his encouragement and guidance and our secretaries and CT technologists for their patience and sense of humor.

William W. Scott, Jr., M.D.
Donna Magid, M.D.
Elliot K. Fishman, M.D.

Contents

Computed Tomography of the Musculoskeletal System

1 Soft Tissue Masses

WILLIAM W. SCOTT, JR.
ELLIOT K. FISHMAN

Very early in the clinical application of CT scanning it became evident that this imaging modality would have considerable usefulness in the evaluation of soft tissue masses. Prior to CT the primary methods for investigation of the soft tissue mass had been plain radiography, xeroradiography, angiography, and ultrasound examination. Continued experience with CT has confirmed its great clinical utility. In this section, we review the documented strengths of CT in the evaluation of soft tissue masses and point out the few pitfalls that have been discovered. The relationship of CT to other imaging methods is outlined. An optimal method for CT examination of soft tissue masses is suggested. The CT findings in specific types of tumors are exemplified with cases from our own experience.

ADVANTAGES OF CT

Computed tomography is very reliable for confirming the presence or absence of a suspected soft tissue mass. Not infrequently, the impression on physical examination that a soft tissue mass is present turns out to be incorrect. It is very important to be able to exclude a mass reliably in such cases. Several authors have commented on the usefulness of CT in this regard. Levine et al.,[1] in a study of 50 patients with suspected musculoskeletal tumors, reported six patients with a negative CT examination, which halted further diagnostic evaluation. In such instances, the value of CT in saving needless expense and anxiety is obvious. Of course, CT is only valuable in this regard if it is reliable. Failures of CT to detect soft tissue masses have been reported in the literature, but are probably preventable with state-of-the-art equipment and careful technique. In one instance, a 12-mm fibrosarcoma was not detected because the interval between scanning sections was too great.[2] In another study of 25 extremity soft tissue lesions, CT failed to detect five lesions. In one case scar tissue could not be distinguished from recurrent tumor. In four cases no lesion was demonstrated by CT when in fact small tumors from 11 to 30 mm in

1

diameter were present. These lesions caused no anatomical distortion and displayed the same attenuation as the surrounding soft tissue.[3] This study was performed on an earlier model scanner, which may have compromised the quality of the study. The authors do not mention whether intravenous contrast medium was specifically utilized in the four cases of undetected soft tissue masses. These few reported cases of undetected lesions should merely serve as a reminder to utilize optimal technique with contiguous or overlapping sections and appropriate contrast enhancement.

Computed tomography optimally demonstrates the size and extent of a mass in the transverse plane, and its relationship to neighboring structures including nerves, vessels, muscles, and bones. This information is of vital importance in planning an optimal therapeutic approach. In recent years, there has been increased utilization of limb-preserving surgery, rather than amputation in cases of malignant extremity tumors.[4-7] For such surgery to be carried out, the exact extent of the tumor and its relationship to important structures must be known. In cases where it is feasible, the tumor-bearing tissues are removed as a unit including presumably normal tissue to an extent of one tissue plane beyond the confines of the suspected tumor. Muscle groups involved are resected from their insertion to origin including the surrounding fascia.[7] Shiu and co-workers have found that close proximity of the lesion to bone or major vessels results in increased risk of local recurrence. For this reason it may be desirable in certain cases to excise portions of the major vessels and replace them with graft and excise portions of bones along with the soft tissue mass.[7] In cases of sarcoma located in the thigh it is important to show that a tumor is confined to the anterior, medial, or posterior compartment or that it is extracompartmental. The latter location has an unfavorable prognosis.[7] CT optimally defines the compartmental anatomy of the thigh.

Computed tomography demonstrates soft tissue masses by distortion of normal architecture or by alteration in the attenuation of the involved tissue. Most authors have found that intravenous contrast enhancement increases the detectability of soft tissue masses by CT.[3,8-10] The margins of muscle groups are generally well visualized by CT due to the small amounts of intervening fat between the different muscle groups. This is almost always true in the thigh and buttocks region, which happens to be the most common location of soft tissue tumors. The vascular structures are generally well outlined by CT with contrast enhancement. Several investigators indicate that optimal enhancement is achieved with a contrast infusion or bolus injection into the veins of the involved extremity during the CT examination.[3,9-11] Because of the axial section of CT, the relationship of a soft tissue mass to the bone is well delineated. It is interesting to note that in one large series[12] actual invasion of the bone by a soft tissue tumor was a relatively rare occurrence. In general, the soft tissue mass merely lies near to the bone or touches the bone without invasion. According to the principles of wide soft part resection surgery described previously, such close contact may necessitate removal of a portion of the bone. The exact operative manipulations may differ; some surgeons merely do a subperiosteal resection and others remove a portion of the bone and replace it with some other material.[7,10] Whatever the operative procedure, CT provides the necessary imaging data. Although this is rare, soft tissue tumors will sometimes invade the bone and the medullary canal of the bone. CT has been shown to demonstrate such tumor invasion.[13]

Since most current scanners have a digital survey view capability, it is possible to reproduce accurately the same axial plane section on follow-up examinations. This feature combined with the excellent display of the extent of a tumor in cross section by CT permits accurate objective follow-up of the response of lesions to chemotherapy, radiotherapy, or surgery.[14] Further discussion of the use of CT in the therapeutic management of patients with soft tissue tumors is found in Chapter 3.

POTENTIAL PITFALLS

Computed tomography has remarkably few limitations in the imaging of soft tissue masses. As previously mentioned, occasional isodense masses are reported which are small, cause no distortion of muscle bundle anatomy, and are thus undetected on CT examination. With optimal contrast enhancement including rapid infusion of contrast followed by sequential bolus injections, the chances of this occurring are slight.

A number of investigators have reported some difficulty with CT imaging in areas where there is little fat.[8,15,16] The fat provides the natural contrast medium between the muscle groups and is important in determining which muscle groups are involved by a tumor. This problem is generally encountered in the lower leg and forearm. Fortunately, major tumors are less common in these regions.[4,7] However, in the majority of cases the lesions are detected due to a difference in attenuation between the tumor and adjacent normal musculature. In cases where CT of these regions is not definitive, it is possible that ultrasound examination might add additional information.[16] In the forearm, one technique that may prove useful is direct longitudinal scanning as described by Nesbit et al.[17] (Fig. 1-1). Another factor that diminishes the importance of this CT deficiency is the relative frequency with which below-knee lesions are treated by amputation rather than more conservative resection.[4] Below-knee protheses function extremely well.

Due to the axial plane of the CT scan it is more difficult to estimate longitudinal extent of tumor than the cross-sectional extent.[2] In practice, due to the resection of muscle bundles from origin to insertion, this feature may not be of clinical importance. In addition, CT with coronal and sagittal image reconstruction can also prove helpful in these cases.

Another problem noted by some investigators[2,9] is the overestimation of lesion size on CT due to the surrounding edema. This is also a problem with angiography. Surrounding edema is a problem primarily with high-grade sarcomas. In practice, this size overestimation may not be a problem. Histologically, high-grade soft tissue sarcomas are surrounded by a "zone composed of granulation-like mesenchymal proliferations whose characteristics are edema and neovascularity."[4] Tongues of neoplasm often extend into and through this

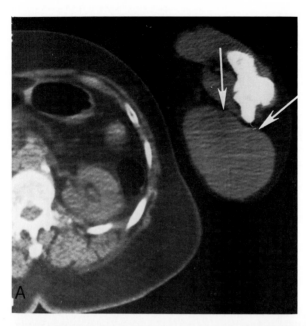

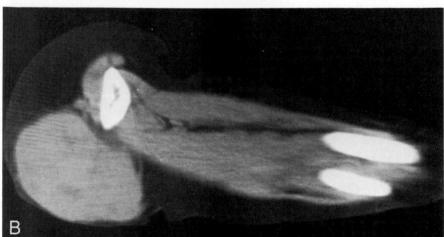

FIG. 1-1. Leiomyosarcoma in a 71-year-old woman with enlarging mass near left elbow. The mass had been present for approximately 4 years. (A) Transaxial CT scan demonstrates large solid mass almost inseparable from muscle at level of elbow joint (arrows). (B) Direct coronal scan demonstrates the full extent of the soft tissue tumor and its relationship to the elbow. At surgery tumor margins were well defined from adjacent normal structures.

zone. Thus it is probably wise to overestimate tumor size if adequate margins are to be achieved.

It is difficult on CT to be certain whether a tumor merely touches or invades the wall of a vessel. For this reason investigators[1,8,9] often recommend angiography if there is an uncertainty about the exact nature of vascular involvement and in cases where prosthetic replacement of vessels is planned. Angiography may be indicated when there is a question about the adequacy of the blood supply to the lower extremities in elderly patients who are undergoing major resections[8] and in patients in whom embolization and intra-arterial chemotherapy are contemplated.[5,8]

Computed tomography frequently demonstrates the sciatic nerve when it is normally surrounded by fat. In cases with a tumor mass near the nerve or with muscles distorted in such a manner that they displace the nerve, involvement of the nerve by tumor usually cannot be determined by CT.[10,12]

Despite these few deficiencies of CT as an imaging modality, it is widely recognized as the procedure of choice for examining soft tissue tumors. In most cases, an imaging work-up should consist of plain radiography, which is the most sensitive method for detecting bony abnormalities, followed by CT examination of the suspected soft tissue mass. It will be interesting to see if magnetic resonance imaging studies will overcome some of the deficiencies of CT.

In general, we do not recommend the use of ultrasound in addition to CT. Some occasions when ultrasound might be employed include masses in the forearm and calf, which are difficult to image due to lack of fat tissue, and repeated follow-up examinations of a tumor mass under treatment. In the latter instance, ultrasound examination might effect a considerable cost saving, while still accurately estimating the tumor volume.

Angiography should be reserved for those cases in which the vessels are inadequately imaged on CT, or those questionably involved by tumor. Angiography will probably be requested by the surgeon prior to surgery with vascular resection and replacement.

METHOD OF EXAMINATION

Examination is usually performed with the patient in a supine position, although the prone position may be advantageous when a lesion is in the gluteal region, to avoid the distortion of the soft tissues in this region and to minimize discomfort to the patient.[8] The patient should be positioned with care so that sections are through the same cephalocaudad level on both sides, allowing symmetry to be utilized in analyzing the images. In addition to the physical examination, a digital radiographic survey film is useful in selecting the region to be examined. Contiguous 8-mm to 1-cm sections should be made from one end of the suspect region to the other including obviously normal regions, both above and below the lesion. The examination should be conducted with intravenous contrast medium enhancement preferably using a constant infusion into a distal vein in the involved extremity during the scanning. If there is a problem with definition of vascular structures, a bolus injection and dynamic sequence of CT scans can be utilized to clarify this anatomy.

In selected cases of forearm involvement, it may be useful to try the direct longitudinal scanning technique mentioned above.[17] In cases where bone involvement appears likely on the standard soft tissue windows, optimal bone imaging windows should be employed to evaluate better the skeletal structures.

To optimize lesion detection, several technical factors should be remembered. (1) Scans should be obtained at a higher mAs station to get better definition of muscle planes. We routinely image the musculoskeletal system at 5.2 sec, 450 mAs, 120 kVp, and 4 mm collimation as opposed to our standard techniques of 3.2 sec, 230 mAs, 120 kVp, and 8 mm collimation. (2) Scans are reviewed and filmed at both standard soft tissue settings (WW-426, WC 21) and with a narrowed window width (WW-140, WC-43). The narrower window width helps to define subtle differences in tissue attenuation.

SPECIFIC LESIONS AND DIFFERENTIAL DIAGNOSIS

In this section we describe the CT appearance of the more common and important soft tissue masses reported in the literature and illustrated from our own experience. In a number of instances such as lipomas, hemangiomas, synovial

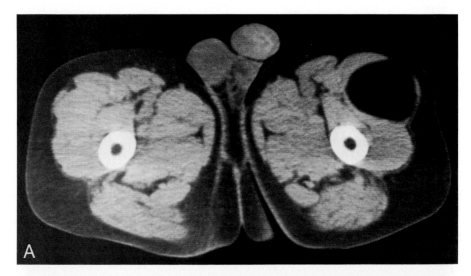

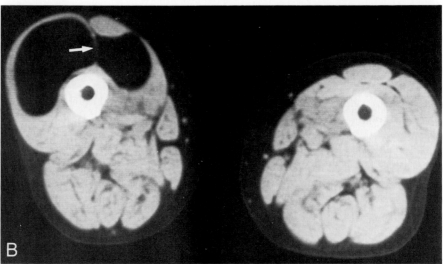

FIG. 1-2. Lipomas in a series of scans from patients with clinically palpable masses. CT was obtained to help determine the cause of the masses. (A) Lipoma (−110 HU) in vastus lateralis muscle. (B) Bilobed lipoma in anterior compartment of thigh. Intramuscular septum is seen (arrow).

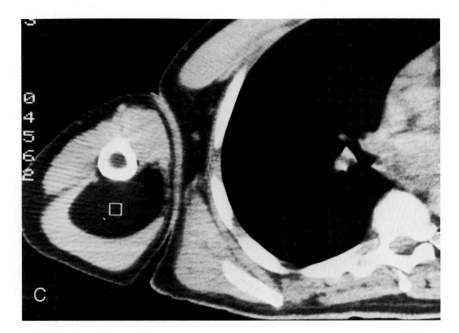

FIG. 1-2. (*Continued*) (C) Mass in posterior portion of right arm. Lipoma is within the vastus lateralis muscle.

cysts, and aneurysm, CT can provide a histologic diagnosis. In a majority of cases, benign and malignant lesions can be differentiated.[12] In contrast to benign lesions, most of the malignant lesions cannot be distinguished from one another.

Benign Lesions

Lipoma

Benign lipoma may be suspected on clinical examination and the diagnosis confirmed by CT in nearly all cases. The lesions are homogeneous, well-defined, and have low CT attenuation (−80 to −130 HU), equivalent to that of subcutaneous fat. There may be some thin streaks of soft tissue running through the lesion, which should not be confused with liposarcoma. Many investigators have been able to diagnose these lesions with confidence[1,2,12,15,16,18-20] (Figs. 1-2, 1-3).

Infiltrative Lipoma

These benign lesions are demonstrated on CT to have a fat content similar to the benign lipoma, but differ in that they have poorly defined margins. They are most common in the lower extremities. Histologically, these legions are known to invade the skeletal muscle locally.[18] Although benign, these are

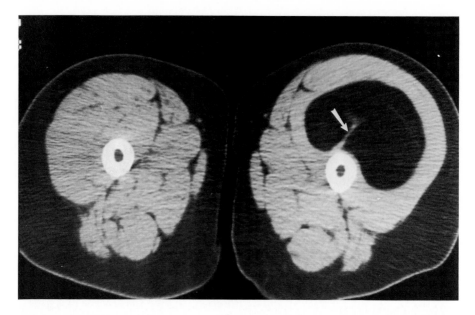

FIG. 1-3. Intramuscular lipoma in a 21-year-old dancer with right thigh pain that had increased over a 3-month period. Clinical diagnosis was sarcoma. A well-defined lipoma is seen in vastus medialis and vastus intermedius. Note the intramuscular septation within the lesion (arrow).

very aggressive lesions and recur in 50 to 60 percent of cases. CT examination is very important to define the extent of these tumors, which is often underestimated. Based solely on the CT appearance, it may be impossible to differentiate between an infiltrating lipoma and a liposarcoma (Figs. 1-4, 1-5). Infiltrating lipomas are often very vascular and may have internal septa that enhance following bolus injection of contrast.

Benign Mesenchymoma of Soft Tissue

These tumors contain two types of mesenchymal tissue not ordinarily found together in addition to fibrous tissue. If a lesion is found to contain definite fat and a large amount of ossification, benign mesenchymoma should be strongly considered. Care should be taken in making this diagnosis as it is a rare lesion.[21] Sometimes these lesions may be named for prominent tissue components, such as "angiolipoma."[18] When these lesions do not contain fat but only ossification, they may be confused with myositis ossificans (Fig. 1-6).

Hemangioma

On CT the hemangioma is generally a well-defined, inhomogeneous lesion. In reported cases[12] round calcifications corresponding to phleboliths have been frequently identified. The finding of such calcifications aids considerably in

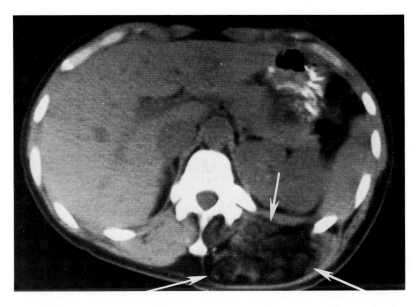

FIG. 1-4. Infiltrating angiomyolipoma in a 34-year-old woman with an enlarging mass on her back. Fatty tumor is seen infiltrating left paraspinal muscles (arrows). Individual muscle bundles can be identified due to fat infiltration.

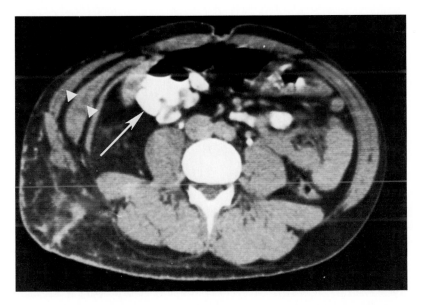

FIG. 1-5. Infiltrating angiolipoma occurring in a 34-year-old man with right flank mass. Tumor infiltrates the anterior abdominal wall musculature separating individual muscle bundles (arrowheads). Tumor extends through the abdominal wall into the abdomen. The ascending colon is displaced medially (arrow).

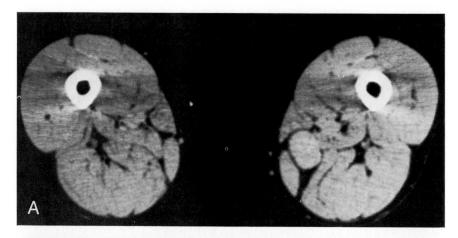

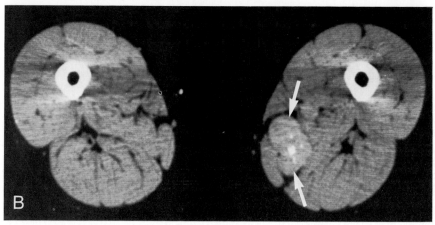

FIG. 1-6. Low-grade mesenchymal tumor presenting in a 42-year-old man as a mass in inner portion of left thigh; it had been present for nearly 2 years. Well-circumscribed mass (arrows) is visible between adductor magnus and gracilis muscles. Speckled calcifications within mass are clearly seen.

making this diagnosis. The lesion shows striking contrast enhancement following rapid bolus injection (Fig. 1-7). Differentiation from arteriovenous malformation may be difficult.

Neural Tumors

A tumor of neural origin such as a schwannoma or neurinoma can be suspected when a major nerve such as the sciatic nerve is seen to enter the center of a mass lesion (Fig. 1-8). Frequently these lesions are of low attenuation and are well defined.[22] Multiple neural tumors may be seen in patients with neuro-

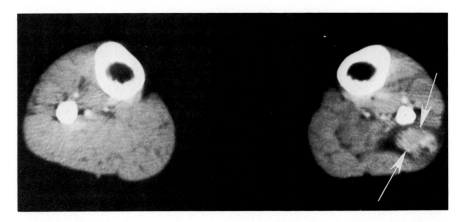

FIG. 1-7. Intramuscular cavernous hemangioma in the left calf of a 21-year-old woman. An enhancing mass (arrows) involves the left soleus muscle. Atrophy of adjacent musculature is also noted, with increasing fat in the intramuscular plane.

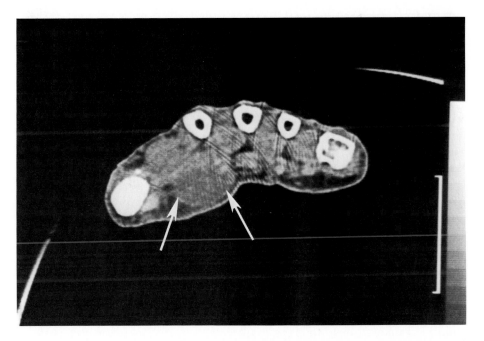

FIG. 1-8. Surgically proven schwannoma of the median nerve presenting in an 88-year-old man as a painful thenar mass. Patient noticed the mass due to difficulty in using cane. Well-demarcated, low-density mass is visible in the course of median nerve (arrows).

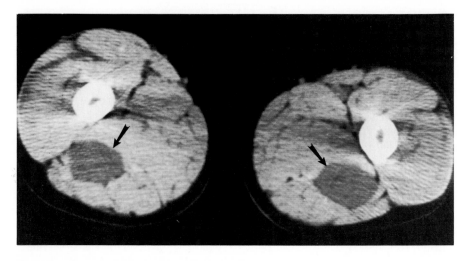

FIG. 1-9. Neurofibromatosis in a 20-year-old man with characteristic clinical stigmata. Bilateral low-density masses (arrows) seen along the course of the sciatic nerve are consistent with neurofibromas. The masses are of lower CT attenuation than muscle, a classic appearance for neurofibromata.

fibromatosis (Fig. 1-9). Plexiform neurofibromas may enhance following injection of contrast material (Fig. 1-10).

Desmoid

Desmoid or aggressive fibromatosis presents as a hypodense or isodense mass that generally becomes hyperdense after intravenous contrast infusion (Fig. 1-11). The margins may be quite poorly defined, and these lesions frequently cannot be differentiated from various sarcomas.[23] There has been one reported case of this lesion[23] in which a hypodense lesion became nearly isodense after contrast infusion. If this particular lesion is suspected, it might be advisable to take several precontrast sections through the area of the lesion to avoid this potential problem. Despite apparently clear surgical margins, desmoid tumors will often recur. These recurrences are also usually hypervascular.

Myositis Ossificans

Following some instances of trauma, soft tissue ossification may develop. However, in some 40 to 60 percent of the cases there is no recognized history of trauma.[24] In such cases, differentiation from periosteal osteosarcoma may be a problem. In many cases plain film examination is diagnostic, but in problem cases CT is very useful to demonstrate the typical zonal phenomenon seen in myositis ossificans.[24,25] The central portion of the lesion has low attenuation while the periphery is of higher attenuation. Variable amounts of bone are found in the periphery depending on age of the lesion, which takes 6 to 8

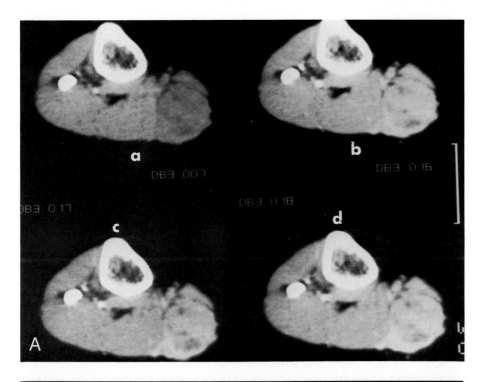

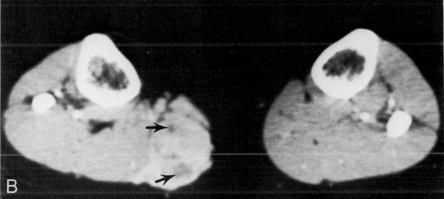

FIG. 1-10.   Plexiform neurofibroma in a 19-year-old woman with a palpable mass in the calf. (A) Sequence of scans pre- and postcontrast enhancement. In image (a) a mass less dense than normal muscle is seen. Following 50 ml bolus of contrast medium via a peripheral vein, marked enhancement of the lesion is seen (images (b) to (d)). Enhancement of lesion is greater than normal muscle. (B) Scan 3 minutes after injection demonstrates enhancement of lesion with areas of central necrosis (arrows).

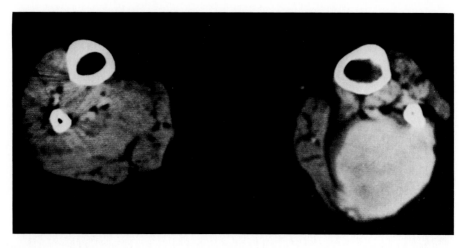

FIG. 1-11.   Desmoid tumor in a 4-year-old girl with mass in left calf. Enhancing tumor infiltrates soleus muscle. Desmoid tumors classically will maintain this enhancement on delayed scans.

weeks to mature. Mature lesions demonstrate a dense shell of bone. These lesions generally do not show a significant mass effect peripheral to the calcification.[19] The central low-attenuation zone corresponds to the undifferentiated, cellular zone seen histologically (Fig. 1-12).

In contrast to myositis ossificans, periosteal sarcoma is more heavily calcified centrally and at its base with a less well defined margin (Fig. 1-13). Dystrophic calcifications in other tumors are usually punctate and do not form a peripheral shell.

Hematoma

The appearance of a soft tissue hematoma is dependent upon its age. Hematomas less than 1 month old usually show areas of both increased and decreased attenuation compared with surrounding soft tissue (Figs. 1-14 to 1-16). A very recent hemorrhage may have strikingly increased attenuation. After approximately 1 month the hematomas usually appear as relatively well-defined, low-attenuation lesions.[19]

Abscess

In the correct clinical setting, the detection on CT of a soft tissue mass containing air bubbles is highly suggestive of an abscess. In most cases abscesses will appear as a low-attenuation soft tissue mass either within muscle or in the subcutaneous tissue. The walls of an abscess often enhance following contrast administration (Fig. 1-17). Detection of abscesses is aided by the use of contrast

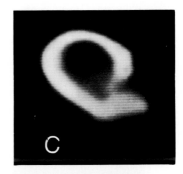

FIG. 1-12. Myositis ossificans in a 12-year-old boy who noted pain in left thigh and a vague history of trauma to the thigh. (A) Plain film of thigh demonstrates soft tissue calcification in lateral portion of thigh (arrow). Notice cortical thickening of the midfemur. (B) Scan through the femur just above the level of calcification demonstrates a water-density mass in the vastus lateralis muscle. An enhancing rim is seen following infusion of intravenous contrast medium (arrows). (C) Image of femur at wide window width shows evidence of prior femoral fracture at level of myositis ossificans.

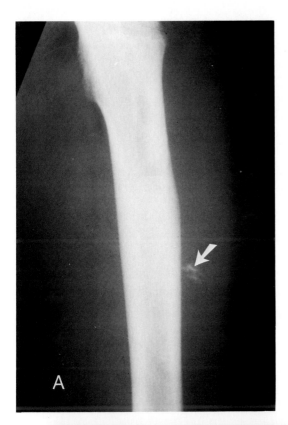

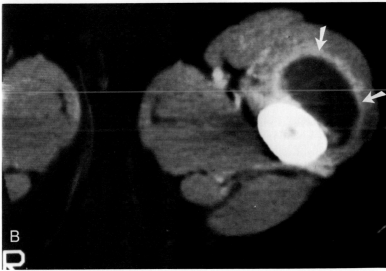

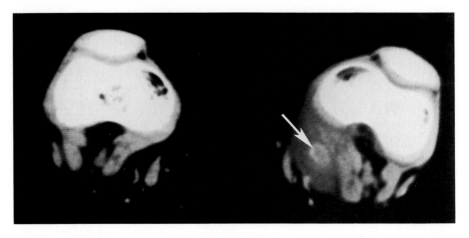

FIG. 1-13. Myositis ossificans in a 5-year-old girl with a palpable mass behind left knee and a vague history of trauma. Soft tissue mass is seen near the medial compartment of the knee joint. Subtle foci of calcification are seen (arrow).

enhancement. Nevertheless, in some cases differentiation from neoplasm is not possible by CT.[12]

Aneurysm

Aneurysm may be suspected by its location along the course of a vessel, especially in the popliteal fossa, and by peripheral rimlike calcification. Luminal enhancement with intravenous contrast administration helps to confirm the diagnosis. In the evaluation of such aneurysms, CT enjoys the same advantage as ultrasound over arteriography, in that it demonstrates the wall of the aneurysm, the clot, and the lumen.[19] If an aneurysm is clinically suspected, ultrasound would be a satisfactory alternative imaging modality (Fig. 1-18).

Synovial Cysts

In the lower extremities synovial cysts are most frequently located adjacent to the knee joint and associated with a knee joint effusion. For this reason the diagnosis should be highly suspect when a well-defined water-density lesion is found near the knee, usually posteriorly, and is associated with a joint effusion. If a synovial cyst is suspected, some investigators advise taking at least one section above the knee through the suprapatellar bursa to evaluate for a knee joint effusion.[19] Diagnosis by CT is rather certain[3,19] but ultrasound examination and arthrography are satisfactory alternative diagnostic methods (Figs. 1-19, 1-20).

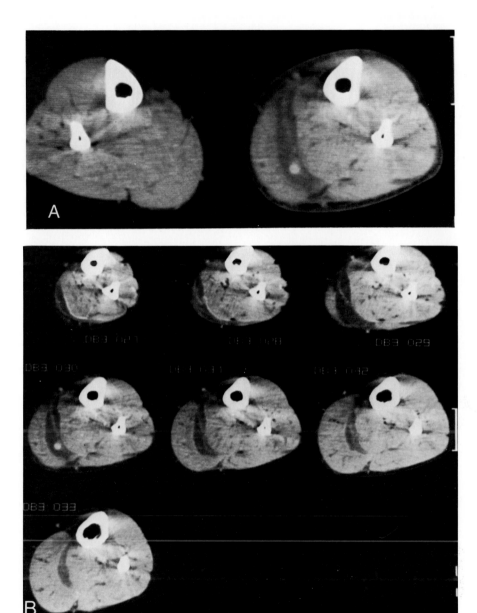

FIG. 1-14. Intramuscular hematoma in a 28-year-old man who experienced pain in the thigh 2 days after vigorous exercise. (A) Low-attenuation zone through gastrocnemius muscle is due to muscle rupture with hematoma. (B) Sequential scans demonstrate full extent of muscle rupture and associated hematoma.

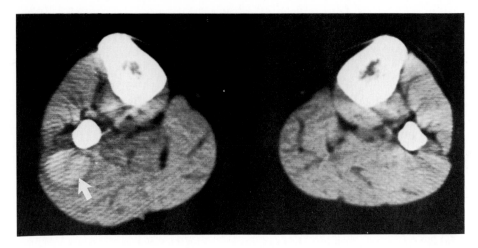

FIG. 1-15. Hematoma in the right calf of a 25-year-old man with Factor VIII deficiency who developed pain and swelling in calf. Hematoma is noted (arrow) in lateral portion of right calf. CT attenuation of hematoma was 70 HU; normal muscle attenuation is 35 HU.

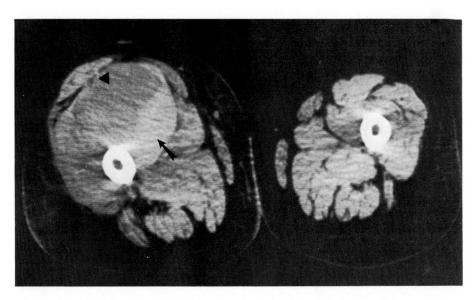

FIG. 1-16. Intramuscular hematoma in a 24-year-old drug addict who experienced pain in right thigh and denied local injection of drugs. Marked swelling of vastus medialis, lateralis, and intermedius is noted. Areas of both high (arrow) and low (arrow-head) CT attenuation are noted, consistent with hematoma.

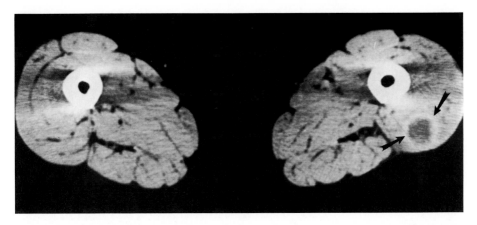

FIG. 1-17. Intramuscular abscess in a 45-year-old man with acquired immune deficiency syndrome (AIDS) and pain in left thigh. A low-density mass with an enhancing rim is seen in the vastus lateralis muscle (arrows). Biopsy of lesion confirmed it to be a staphylococcal abscess.

Malignant Lesions

Liposarcoma

Liposarcoma is probably the most common malignant soft tissue sarcoma. In the M.D. Anderson series of 499 consecutive soft tissue sarcomas, 21 percent were liposarcoma.[26] Five histologic types are recognized: differentiated, embryonal, myxoid, pleomorphic, and round cell. These tumors consist of admixtures of fat cells and soft tissue components in varying proportions. The CT attenuation depends on the relative amounts of fat and soft tissue densities admixed. For this reason, some of the lesions with relatively high fat content can be recognized as distinct from other sarcomatous tumors. There is some suggestion that a relatively high fat content and, hence, a low attenuation, may correlate with the better-differentiated tumors with a better prognosis.[8,18] deSantos et al.,[26] in a series of 17 cases of liposarcoma, were able to make a specific diagnosis by CT in only four cases utilizing the fatty nature of the tumor. These investigators believe that an attenuation of −20 HU or lower is necessary to differentiate fat from necrotic tumor tissue, which might mimic an area of fat. In some of these tumors of higher grade, the margins may be ill-defined. The fact that CT cannot define the tumor type is not a particular disadvantage. In most cases, the role of CT is to determine the extent of the tumor, which is done quite accurately. In one study of 77 patients with soft tissue sarcomas, CT correctly predicted operability in 22 of 24 patients[11] (Figs. 1-21 to 1-24).

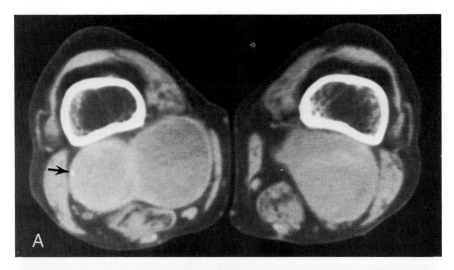

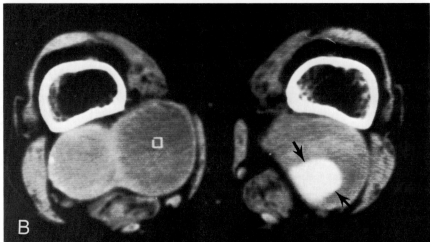

FIG. 1-18. Popliteal artery aneurysm in a 70-year-old man with a palpable mass in the posterior compartment of right knee. (A) Non-contrast-enhanced study demonstrates cystic masses in both posterior knee compartments. Note calcification in the wall of mass on right (arrow). (B) Following infusion of contrast medium the lumen of the popliteal artery enhances (arrows). Notice displacement of adjacent muscle bundles without direct involvement.

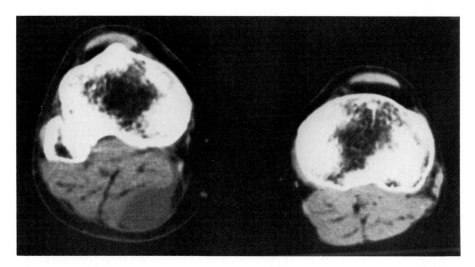

FIG. 1-19. Synovial cyst in a 52-year-old man with recent onset of left knee pain and limp. Fluid-filled mass is seen posterior to semitendinosus muscle, compatible with synovial cyst.

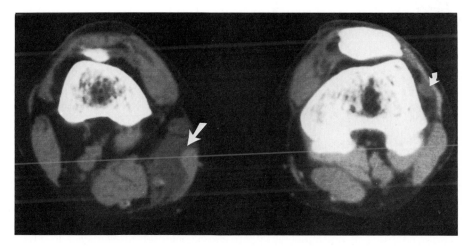

FIG. 1-20. Synovial cysts in a 37-year-old man with persistent knee pain following ski accident. Bilateral synovial cysts are seen (arrows). Notice that synovial cysts may be found in various locations near the joint space.

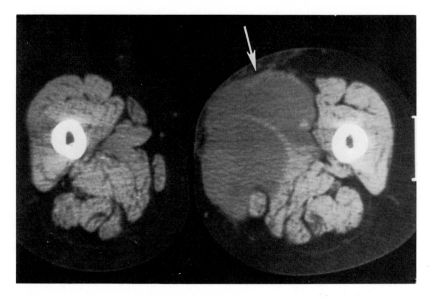

FIG. 1-21. Liposarcoma in a 45-year-old woman who experienced a painful mass in her left thigh. Low-density mass (5 HU) infiltrates the gracilis and adductor muscles. The tumor appears to infiltrate the subcutaneous tissues (arrow).

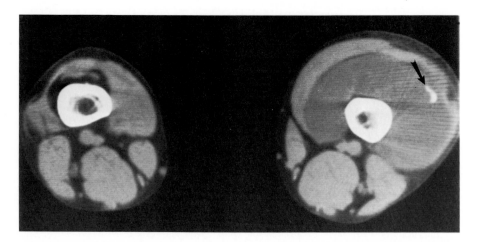

FIG. 1-22. Liposarcoma in a 29-year-old man with painful mass in left thigh. Extensive tumor involving the anterior compartment of the thigh is seen. The mass is of low CT attenuation (−10 HU—+10 HU). Foci of dystrophic calcification are also noted (arrow).

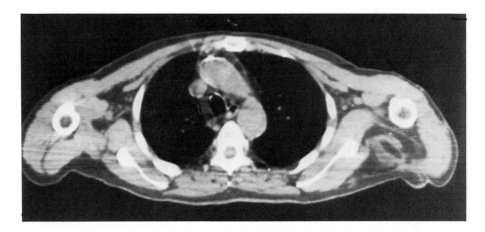

FIG. 1-23. Liposarcoma in a 75-year-old man who presented with a painful swelling of the left shoulder and axilla. Fatty tumor is infiltrating muscles of the shoulder with central linear densities commonly seen in liposarcoma. No underlying bony involvement is noted.

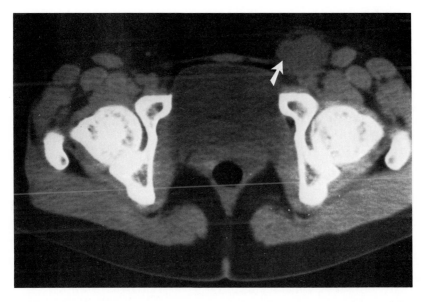

FIG. 1-24. Liposarcoma in a 32-year-old woman who noted an enlarging left groin mass. Soft tissue mass is seen (arrow) in the left inguinal region displacing the sartorius muscle. Tumor is of low CT attenuation but not of fatty density.

Fibrosarcoma and Malignant Fibrous Histiocytoma

In the majority of cases, soft tissue sarcomas have an attenuation range of −20 to 50 HU, which is significantly lower than the adjacent muscle. The only exception to this is the occasional liposarcoma with significant proportions of fat, as mentioned above.[2,11,26] The margins of these tumors may be ill-defined and there has been some difficulty in estimating extent of the tumor due to surrounding edema, which causes an overestimation (Fig. 1-25). In general, sarcomas such as fibrosarcoma and malignant fibrous histiocytoma (MFH) are more homogeneous than the liposarcoma[2] (Fig. 1-26). CT may demonstrate small dystrophic calcifications in MFH that are usually not detected on standard x-ray studies.

Soft Tissue Chondrosarcoma

Several cases of soft tissue chondrosarcoma have been reported. This is an unusual tumor, but it may be identified by the prominent calcifications which typically occur. Whenever a soft tissue mass with calcification is encountered, this lesion should be considered along with possible soft tissue osteosarcoma or calcification in metastatic disease, such as mucinous adenocarcinoma.[2,27] Many types of soft tissue sarcomas, including rhabdomyosarcomas and poorly differentiated sarcomas, show small areas of dystrophic calcification (Fig. 1-27).

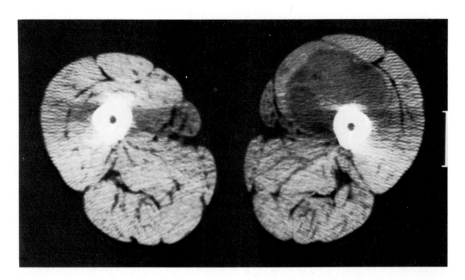

FIG. 1-25. Malignant fibrous histiocytoma presented in a 45-year-old man as fullness and pain in the thigh. A mass infiltrating the vastus medialis and intermedius is seen. The mass is of lower attenuation than muscle (20 HU) but is not of fat density. Narrowing of window width helps to define the lesion better.

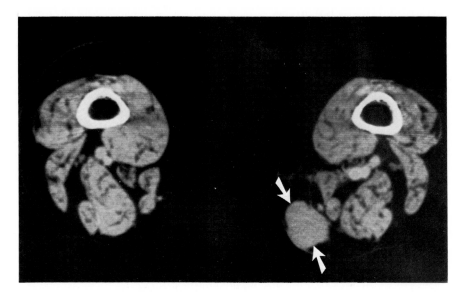

FIG. 1-26. Malignant fibrous histiocytoma in a 61-year-old woman presented as a mass above the medial portion of the knee. Solid tumor is clearly defined in subcutaneous fat (arrows). The mass is slightly denser than normal muscle and did not enhance following infusion of contrast medium.

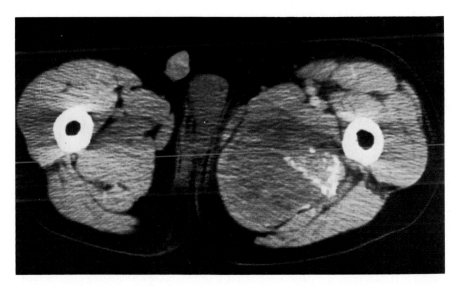

FIG. 1-27. Rhabdomyosarcoma in a 28-year-old woman who noted a mass in her left thigh. The mass involves vastus medialis muscle of lower attenuation than normal muscle. Multiple foci of calcification are also noted.

ACKNOWLEDGMENT

We gratefully acknowledge the contributions of the Johns Hopkins Tumor Registry and the assistance of Mrs. Joyce Kane and Ms. Anne Kammer.

REFERENCES

1. Levine E, Lee KR, Neff JR et al: Comparison of computed tomography and other imaging modalities in the evaluation of musculoskeletal tumors. Radiology 131:431, 1979
2. Egund N, Ekelund L, Sako M et al: CT of soft-tissue tumors. AJR 137:725, 1981
3. Bernardino ME, Jing B, Thomas JL et al: The extremity soft-tissue lesion: a comparative study of ultrasound, computed tomography, and xeroradiography. Radiology 139:53, 1981
4. Enneking WF, Spanier SS, Malawer MM: The effect of the anatomic setting on the results of surgical procedures for soft parts sarcoma of the thigh. Cancer 47:1005, 1981
5. Morton DL, Eilber FR, Townsend CM et al: Limb salvage from a multidisciplinary treatment approach for skeletal and soft tissue sarcomas of the extremity. Ann Surg 184:268, 1976
6. Fortner JG, Kim DK, Shiu MH: Limb-preserving vascular surgery for malignant tumors of the lower extremity. Arch Surg 112:391, 1977
7. Shiu MH, Castro EB, Steven IH et al: Surgical treatment of 297 soft tissue sarcomas of the lower extremity. Ann Surg 182:597, 1975
8. Levine E: Computed tomography of musculoskeletal tumors. CRC Crit Rev Diagn Imaging 16:279, 1981
9. Ekelund L, Herrlin K, Rydholm A: Comparison of computed tomography and angiography in the evaluation of soft tissue tumors of the extremities. Acta Radiol Diagn 23:15, 1982
10. Heelan RT, Watson RC, Smith J: Computed tomography of lower extremity tumors. AJR 132:933, 1979
11. Golding SJ, Husband JE: The role of computed tomography in the management of soft tissue sarcomas. Br J Radiol 55:740, 1982
12. Weekes RG, McLeod RA, Reiman HM et al: CT of soft-tissue neoplasms. AJR 144:355, 1985
13. Kagan AR, Steckel RJ: Diagnostic oncology case study: intramedullary extension of a soft-tissue neoplasm. AJR 139:807, 1982
14. Berger PE, Kuhn JP: Computed tomography of tumors of the musculoskeletal system in children. Radiology 127:171, 1978
15. deSantos LA, Goldstein HM, Murray JA et al: Computed tomography in the evaluation of musculoskeletal neoplasms. Radiology 128:89, 1978
16. Yiu-Chiu VS, Chiu LC: Complementary values of ultrasound and computed tomography in the evaluation of musculoskeletal masses. RadioGraphics 3:46, 1983
17. Nesbit D, Levine E, Neff JR: Direct longitudinal computed tomography of the forearm. J Comput Assist Tomogr 5(1):144, 1981
18. Hunter JC, Johnson WH, Genant HK: Computed tomography evaluation of fatty tumors of the somatic soft tissues: clinical utility and radiologic-pathologic correlation. Skel Radiol 4:79, 1979
19. Heiken JP, Lee KT, Smathers RL et al: CT of benign soft-tissue masses of the extremities. AJR 142:575, 1984
20. Wilson JS, Korobkin M, Genant HK et al: Computed tomography of musculoskeletal disorders. AJR 131:55, 1978
21. Hudson TM, Bertoni F, Enneking WF: Computed tomography of a benign mesenchymoma of soft tissue. J Comput Assist Tomogr 9(1):205, 1985
22. Weinberger G, Levinsohn EM: Computed tomography in the evaluation of sarcomatous tumors of the thigh. AJR 130:115, 1978

23. Hudson TM, Vandergriend RA, Springfield DS et al: Aggressive fibromatosis: evaluation by computed tomography and angiography. Radiology 150:495, 1984
24. Zeanah WR, Hudson TM: Myositis ossificans: radiologic evaluation of two cases with diagnostic computed tomograms. Clin Orthop 168:187, 1982
25. Amendola MA, Glazer GM, Agha FP et al: Myositis ossificans circumscripta computed tomographic diagnosis. Radiology 149:775, 1983
26. deSantos LA, Ginaldi S, Wallace S: Computed tomography in liposarcoma. Cancer 47:46, 1981
27. Hermann G, Yeh H, Schwartz I: Computed tomography of soft-tissue lesions of the extremities, pelvic and shoulder girdles: sonographic and pathological correlations. Clin Radiol 35:193, 1984

2 Primary Bone Tumors

RICHARD P. MOSER, JR.

This chapter demonstrates the importance of CT in the evaluation of benign and malignant primary bone tumors. Since primary bone tumors are rare, any suspected malignant skeletal neoplasm (especially in an adult) is due to metastases, lymphoma, or myeloma, until proven otherwise. Metastases are most easily excluded by correlation with clinical history and nuclear medicine bone scan.

CLASSIFICATION OF BONE TUMORS

Prior to directing attention to the role of CT in the evaluation of primary bone tumors, it is necessary to establish a classification of skeletal neoplasms. One useful classification is based on the tissue of origin of the tumor, to include benign and malignant counterparts: (1) cartilage: benign—enchondroma, osteochondroma, chondroblastoma, chondromyxoidfibroma; malignant—chondrosarcoma; (2) bone: benign—osteoma, osteoid osteoma, osteoblastoma; malignant—osteosarcoma; (3) fibrous connective tissue: benign—desmoplastic fibroma, cortical desmoid; malignant—fibrosarcoma; (4) marrow tissues: benign—lipoma; malignant—myeloma, Ewing's sarcoma or other round cell lesions, liposarcoma; (5) vascular: benign—angioma, lymphangioma; malignant—angiosarcoma.[1]

This is but one simplified approach to a classification of primary benign and malignant skeletal neoplasms. Additional entities to consider (but more difficult to place easily in the preceding classification) include bone cyst, fibroxanthoma, aneurysmal bone cyst, adamantinoma, giant cell tumor (osteoclastoma), glomus tumor, hemangiopericytoma, malignant fibrous histiocytoma, or multiple lesions (such as diffuse fibromatosis, multiple enchondromatosis, multiple osteochondromatosis, or multiple angiomatosis). Furthermore, atten-

The opinions or assertions contained herein are the private views of the author and are not to be construed as official or as reflecting the views of the Department of the Army or the Department of Defense.

tion must also be directed toward the epicenter of the lesion, since malignant bone tumors that arise within or invade the medullary shaft of the bone usually have a worse prognosis than those that arise on the surface of the bone and grow outward (parosteal or periosteal tumors). To make the classification more complete, it is necessary to recall that most benign bone tumors can undergo malignant transformation, although this occurs in only a small percentage of cases. Even nontumorous conditions such as Paget's disease and bone infarction may occasionally be complicated by malignant transformation.

The plain radiograph is used to determine (1) which part of the bone is affected: diaphysis, metaphysis, or epiphysis; (2) the appearance of the margins of the lesion: well-defined geographic destruction with or without sclerotic margins (low biologic activity), moth-eaten destruction (intermediate biologic activity), or permeative destruction (fastest growth, most active biologically);[2] (3) the appearance of the periosteal response of the tumor; again, an indication of the biological activity of the lesion;[3] and (4) the appearance of the matrix of the lesion: solid, cloud-like, or ivory-like matrix indicating mineralized osteoid; stippled, flocculent, or ring and arc mineralization indicating a cartilage matrix; or a nonmineralized matrix.[4] Ischemic ossification and dystrophic mineralization can have stippled, flocculent, or even a patchy solid density pattern. In each of these situations, CT is complementary to plain film radiography in the evaluation of bone tumors. Rarely, if ever, is the CT alone diagnostic.

After plain radiography establishes a differential diagnosis, CT should be performed prior to biopsy or definitive surgery. This chapter illustrates the additional diagnostic information to be gained by the use of CT.

IMPORTANCE OF COMPUTED TOMOGRAPHY

Detecting Obscure Lesions

CT is invaluable in detecting bone tumors in the pelvis where overlying bowel gas and feces can obscure the bony detail on the routine radiograph. Bone tumors in the vertebral column also may be readily apparent on CT when still difficult to detect on a plain radiograph.[5] Areas of the skeleton that are most difficult to image on plain radiographs are frequently best imaged by CT. Figures 2-1 and 2-2 illustrate the utility of CT in anatomically difficult areas.

Determining the Extent of the Lesion

CT is far superior to plain radiography for evaluating the size and extent of the lesion, especially in flat bones such as the pelvis and scapula (Fig. 2-3). Subtle pathologic fracture or cortical disruption is best detected by CT (Figs. 2-4, 2-5). The extent of periosteal reaction is clearly evident on CT. The relationship of the tumor to adjacent soft tissue structures is extremely important and is best accomplished with CT. Naturally, invasion of muscle groups or

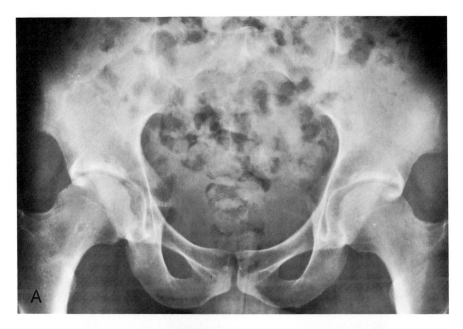

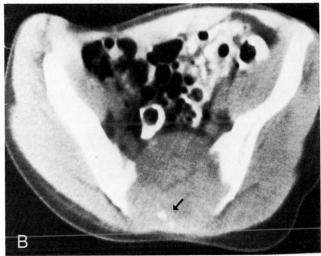

FIG. 2-1.   Giant cell tumor in a 30-year-old man who had had back pain for 6 months. (A) Anteroposterior radiograph of the pelvis shows a large amount of bowel gas and feces obscuring the sacrum. (B) CT scan detects the obscure lesion: a large lytic lesion of the sacrum is noted with some extension of the tumor into the adjacent anterior and posterior soft tissues. A faint amount of mineralization is noted in the lesion (arrow). The age of the patient, location of the tumor, and predominantly nonmineralized matrix are consistent with giant cell tumor of bone. (Case courtesy of Jack Edeiken, M.D., Professor and Chairman, Department of Radiology, Thomas Jefferson University Hospital, Philadelphia, PA.)

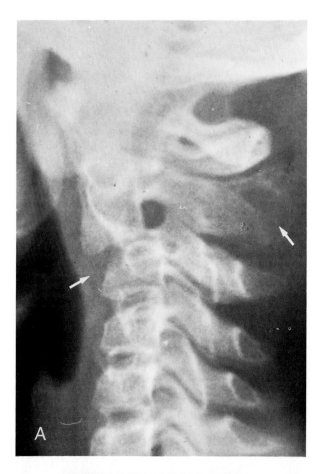

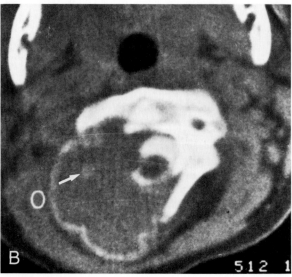

FIG. 2-2. Osteoblastoma of the cervical spine in a 7-year-old girl with pain and swelling in the neck. (A) Lateral radiograph of the cervical spine shows an interesting anterior subluxation of C2 with regard to C3 (long arrow) and widening of the posterior elements of C2 (short arrow). (B) CT scan determines extent of the lesion and subtle matrix mineralization. CT allows much better definition of anatomic detail. Metrizamide is noted within a slightly deformed spinal sac. There is a large "expansile" lesion originating from the right side posterior elements of C2, with some very faint mineralization (arrow) within the tumor on the CT scan. This subtle mineralization could not be appreciated on plain films. The location of the lesion as well as the combined plain film and CT findings (especially the subtle matrix mineralization) are consistent with the diagnosis of osteoblastoma.

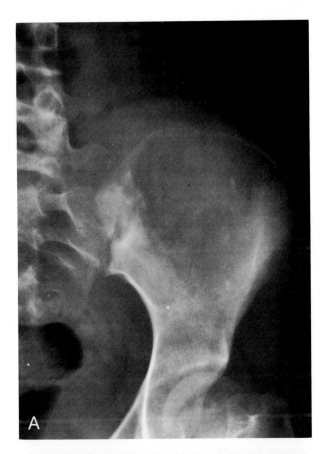

FIG. 2-3. Ewing's sarcoma in a 12-year-old girl with intermittent hip pain for 1 month. (A) Anteroposterior radiograph of the left ilium shows a large ill-defined lytic lesion with associated soft tissue mass. The relationship of the lesion to the left sacroiliac joint and the epicenter of the lesion is unclear. (B) CT scan determines extent and epicenter of the lesion. The CT scan clearly shows that the lesion begins inside the ilium and extends into the adjacent soft tissue. A huge soft tissue mass is noted both in the pelvis and, to a lesser extent, in the buttocks region (arrowheads). The relationship of the lesion to the adjacent sacroiliac joint is best appreciated on CT. Mineralization is not a predominant finding on the CT scan. The age of the patient, location of the tumor, and correlation of the radiograph and the CT are all consistent with Ewing's sarcoma.

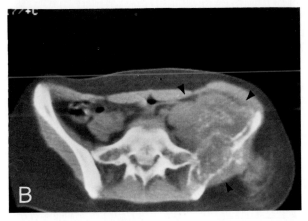

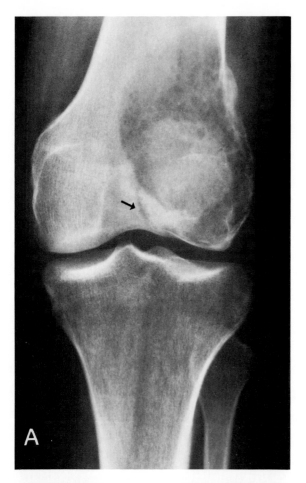

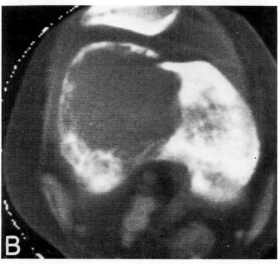

FIG. 2-4. Giant cell tumor presenting in a 26-year old woman with knee pain and episodes of "giving way" and falling. (A) An AP radiograph of the knee shows an eccentric lytic lesion in the distal femur with extension close to the articular surface. There is some lateral cortical irregularity. A subtle fracture extending to the articular surface is also seen (arrow). (B) A CT scan assesses the matrix of the lesion and demonstrates discontinuity of the anterior femoral cortex. In addition, there is no significant mineralization of the matrix of this large lesion that occupies the entire lateral condyle of the distal femur. The age of the patient, the location of the lesion in the distal femur, the plain radiographic findings of eccentric epicenter and extension toward the subarticular area, and the predominantly nonmineralized matrix are all consistent with giant cell tumor.

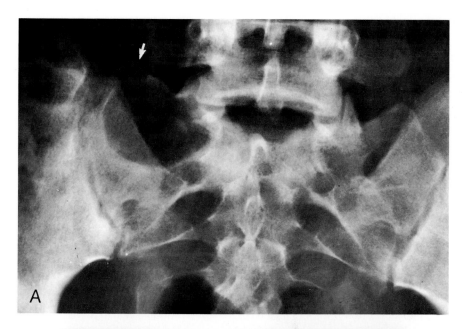

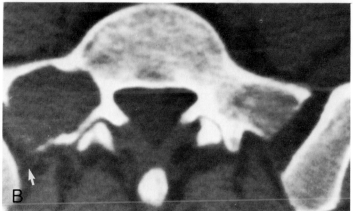

FIG. 2-5.   Chondromyxoidfibroma in a 17-year-old girl with a 6-month history of pain localized to the region of the right sacroiliac joint. (A) A geographic lytic lesion with sclerotic margin is noted in the right wing of the sacrum (arrow) on an AP radiograph of the sacrum. (B) The CT scan assesses the matrix and the extent of the lesion and demonstrates that the lesion arises within the sacrum; there is a nonmineralized matrix. The posterior cortex is irregular, suggesting pathologic fracture (arrow). For reasons that are poorly understood, the matrix of chondromyxoidfibroma rarely mineralizes.

adjacent neurovascular structures can drastically alter the contemplated surgery. If there is mineralization of the tumor matrix, CT can best assess the extent of involvement of the medullary canal. This assessment can have significant therapeutic implications, such as determining the length of required curettage of a benign bone tumor or the level of amputation in a malignant bone tumor of the distal forearm or distal lower leg. If the tumor matrix is *not* mineralized, determining the extent of medullary shaft involvement by CT is more hazardous and considerably less reliable. Because of its greater discrimination of subtle density differences, CT is superior to plain radiography in detecting early or faint matrix mineralization that might not be appreciated on the plain film. Detection of such subtle matrix mineralization would alter the list of favored differential diagnoses. CT can also detect distant metastases of malignant bone tumors.[6,7]

Assessing the Matrix of the Bone Tumor

A nonmineralized matrix suggests giant cell tumor, fibrocystic lesions, or malignant fibrous histiocytoma.[8] Stippled, flocculent, or rings-and-arcs mineralization suggests cartilage lesions (Figs. 2-6, 2-7) (although the matrices of chondroblastoma and chondromyxoidfibroma rarely mineralize).[9-19] Solid, cloud-like, or ivory-like confluent mineralization suggests osteoblastoma or osteosarcoma[20] (Fig. 2-8). These are, however, generalizations. For example, occasionally the osteoblastoma does not mineralize and the osteosarcoma is markedly osteolytic. Usually the correct diagnosis (or reasonable differential diagnosis) of the bone tumor is anticipated from the plain radiograph, but subtle tumor matrix mineralization apparent only on CT can be invaluable in establishing the correct diagnosis.

Detecting the Epicenter of the Lesion

Computed tomography is extremely sensitive in determining the epicenter of the lesion. It is important to know whether the lesion is primarily of soft tissue or bony origin.[21-23] Large masses involving the chest wall, for instance, may be of soft tissue or bone (i.e., rib) origin, a distinction that often is not readily apparent on plain radiographs (Figs. 2-9 to 2-11). Furthermore, an incorrect diagnosis can be made if the lesion is not biopsied at its origin. For instance, an osteosarcoma that originates in the tibia but breaks through the cortex into the adjacent soft tissue can demonstrate histologic findings consistent with osteosarcoma, chondrosarcoma, pleomorphic sarcoma, or a combination of cell types if biopsied in its extraosseous soft tissue extent. If the only viable therapy for the malignant bone tumor is amputation, failure to use CT and biopsy the lesion at its site of origin might be unimportant. However, if meaningful data are ever to be derived from varying surgical, chemotherapeutic, and/or radiation therapy treatment protocols, the correct diagnosis is critical to preclude erroneous conclusions concerning the success or failure of differing treatments.

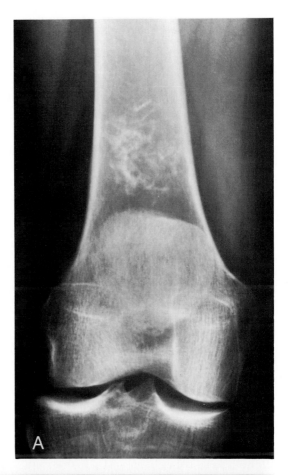

FIG. 2-6. Enchondroma of the distal femur in a 53-year-old woman with pain after twisting her knee. (A) Curvilinear and flocculent mineralization is seen in the distal diaphysis on an AP radiograph of the distal femur. There is no evidence of cortical disruption. (B) The CT scan assesses the matrix and the extent of the lesion and demonstrates no evidence of cortical disruption or adjacent soft tissue involvement. The curvilinear mineralization pattern is typical of that encountered in mineralized cartilage matrix. The plain radiographic and CT findings, particularly with regard to central distal femoral diaphyseal location and the pattern of mineralization, are consistent with enchondroma.

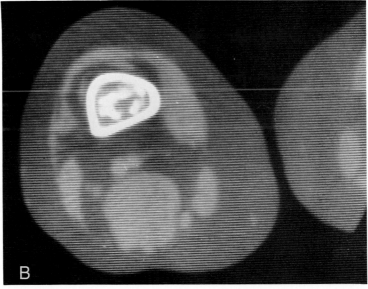

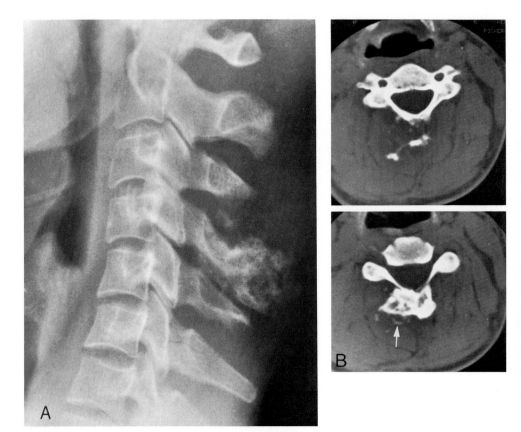

FIG. 2-7. Chondrosarcoma of the cervical spine in a 35-year-old woman with neck stiffness, pain, and an associated palpable mass. (A) Lateral radiograph of the cervical spine shows a lesion of the spinous process of C4 with some adjacent soft tissue mineralization. (B) CT scan assesses the matrix and the extent of the lesion. The lesion begins within the spinous process and is mixed lytic/blastic. There is evidence of curvilinear mineralization within the adjacent soft tissues (arrow), the pattern of which suggests mineralized cartilage matrix. Indistinct margins and soft tissue involvement on the radiograph and CT are signs of potential malignancy. (Case courtesy of Jack Edeiken, M.D., Professor and Chairman, Department of Radiology, Thomas Jefferson University Hospital, Philadelphia, PA.)

Determing the Relationship of Tumor to Cortex of the Involved Bone

Computed tomography shows the relationship of the bone tumor to the surface of the bone and shows whether the growth is completely exophytic or whether there is penetration into the medullary space.[24-27] Subtle alterations in marrow attenuation imply tumor infiltration and extension. These relationships have important diagnostic and therapeutic implications yet are frequently difficult or impossible to appreciate on plain radiographs (Fig. 2-12). For instance, par-

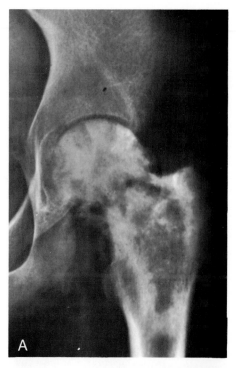

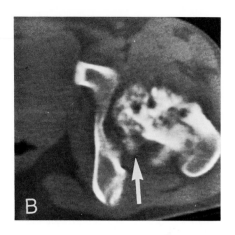

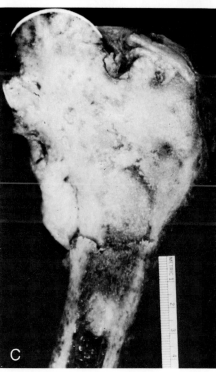

FIG. 2-8. Osteosarcoma of femur presenting in a 17-year-old man with hip pain for 4 months. (A) On the AP radiograph of the left hip there is a mixed lytic/sclerotic lesion involving the proximal left femur. In an older patient, the radiograph might be confused with Paget's disease (although in Paget's disease other sites of skeletal involvement, including the adjacent acetabulum, would be anticipated). (B) The CT scan assesses the epicenter and the matrix of the lesion and demonstrates that this is a mixed lytic/blastic lesion of intraosseous origin breaking out into the adjacent soft tissue where some mineralization is also noted (arrow). The CT scan does not demonstrate a predominantly cortical disease, thereby excluding Paget's disease. The matrix mineralization is rather confluent and there is no significant evidence of curvilinear mineralization to suggest a chondroid matrix. The plain radiograph and CT are consistent with osteosarcoma. (C) Coronal hemisected gross specimen. The proximal femur is replaced with tumor and there is a skip area of medullary involvement distal to a fracture.

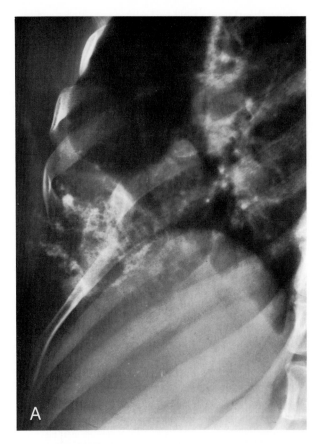

FIG. 2-9. Malignant transformation of enchondroma to chondrosarcoma in a 47-year-old woman with a known abnormal chest radiograph since age 17. She had a 3-year history of increasing chest pain and a history of enchondromatosis. (A) Right rib film shows marked rib destruction with extensive soft tissue mineralization in punctate and arclike configurations. (B) The CT scan provides a better appreciation of the intrathoracic extent of the large right chest mass. The plain radiograph and CT suggest a lesion composed of mineralizing cartilage, probably arising from a lower right rib. The huge soft tissue extension (arrows) suggests malignancy (image filmed with double window technique).

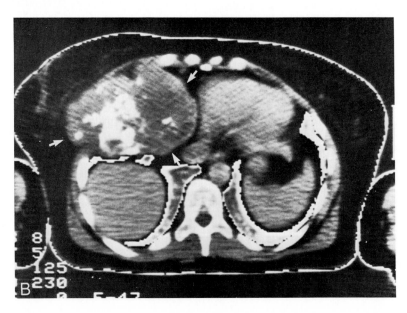

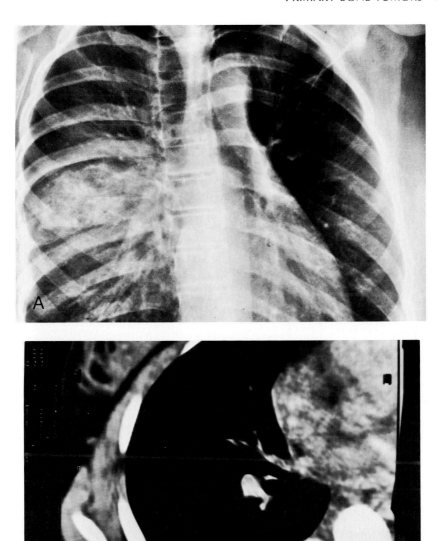

FIG. 2-10.   Osteoblastoma of a rib in a 16-year-old girl with a 1-year history of worsening pain medial to the right scapula. (A) Frontal chest radiograph shows a large area of increased density overlying the right midchest with involvement of the right seventh posterior rib. The site of origin of the lesion cannot be determined. (B) The CT scan clearly demonstrates that the lesion originates in the posterior rib (arrow). There is extensive confluent mineralization throughout the lesion. The plain radiograph and CT are consistent with osteoblastoma.

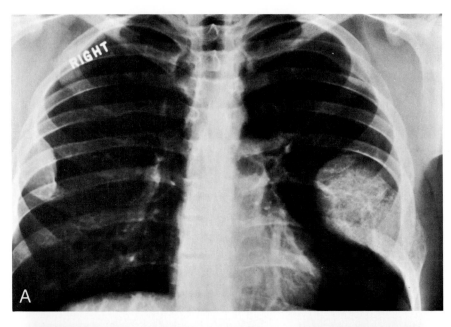

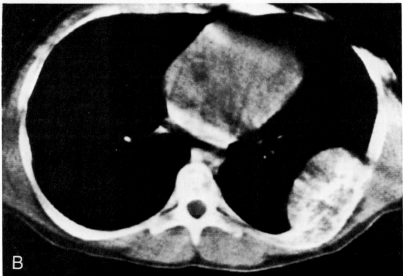

FIG. 2-11. Multiple angiomas of bone in a 14-year-old boy. (A) Routine chest radiograph taken at the time of hospital admission shows large "expansile" lesions involving the left seventh and right fourth ribs. (B) The CT scan demonstrates the epicenter of the lesion within the left seventh rib. There is a linear mineralization pattern. Combined plain radiograph and CT findings are consistent with the diagnosis of angioma of bone.

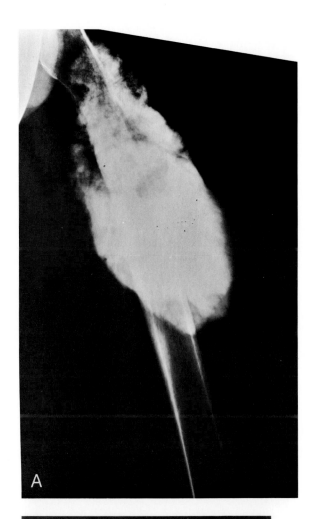

FIG. 2-12. Periosteal sarcoma of the femur in a 15-year-old boy with pain and swelling first noted after mild trauma. (A) On a plain radiograph of the femur, extensive confluent mineralization obscures the proximal shaft of the femur. Due to the large size and the extensive mineralization of the mass, the site of origin cannot be determined from the plain film. (B) CT scan determines the relationship of the lesion to the cortex of the involved bone and demonstrates that the mineralization surrounds the shaft of the femur without an obvious cleavage plain between the mineralization in the lesion and the underlying bone. The findings are consistent with periosteal sarcoma. A subtle increase in medullary cavity attentuation (seen on other CT scans not illustrated here) raised the possibility of intramedullary extension of this periosteal lesion. The plain radiograph and CT are consistent with periosteal sarcoma.

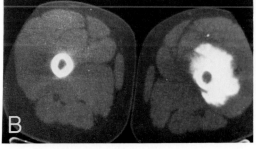

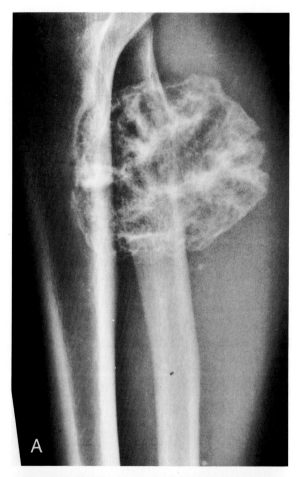

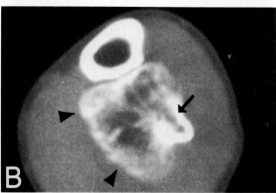

FIG. 2-13. Osteochondroma of the fibula in a 20-year-old man with a firm, nontender, slowly enlarging mass in the popliteal area. (A) Lateral radiograph of the proximal lower leg shows the large lesion overlying the proximal tibia and fibula. There is extensive mineralization involving the lesion. The exact site of origin of the lesion cannot be determined. An incidental small ossified fibroxanthoma is noted in the proximal tibia, best seen on the frontal radiograph, which is not illustrated. (B) CT scan determines the relationship of the lesion to the cortex of the involved bone and clearly demonstrates that the medullary space of the fibula opens into the lesion (arrow). The lesion has a well-defined peripheral margin (arrowheads) and extensive mineralization. The lesion is causing some remodeling compression changes on the adjacent tibial cortex. The plain radiograph and CT are consistent with osteochondroma. (*Figure continues.*)

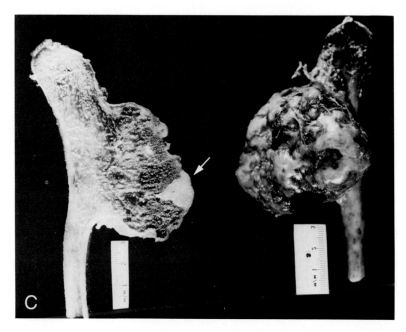

FIG. 2-13. (*Continued*) (C) Gross photograph of both external (right) and cut (left) surfaces of the osteochondroma after resection of the proximal fibula. The transected specimen (left) clearly demonstrates the intramedullary space of the host bone contiguous with that of the lesion (a finding demonstrated clearly on CT). On this same image note the nonuniform thickness of the peripheral cartilage cap, which dips in one area in a triangular fashion toward the center of the lesion (arrow). The external appearance (right) demonstrates the lobular growth pattern typical of a cartilaginous lesion.

osteal osteosarcoma (osteosarcoma arising at the surface of the bone) frequently has a better prognosis than osteosarcoma arising within the medullary canal. Occasionally, although the plain radiograph is consistent with a parosteal sarcoma, the lesion might demonstrate intramedullary penetration appreciable only on CT. The presence of intramedullary involvement would naturally affect the proposed surgery. Furthermore, parosteal sarcoma is most commonly encountered in the distal femur where it can be indistinguishable from a sessile osteochondroma on the plain radiograph. If CT demonstrates the marrow space of the host bone contiguous with that of the lesion arising from its surface, the diagnosis of osteochondroma can be made (Fig. 2-13).

Influencing Management of the Bone Tumor

Computed tomography can affect the management of bone tumors in numerous additional ways, including the following. CT can suggest the best approach for biopsy (the biopsy might be done under CT guidance), perhaps to avoid areas of suspected necrosis (where a definitive diagnosis cannot be made easily) or to aim for areas that were mineralized on earlier scans but are no longer mineralized on the present CT (suggesting increased biologic activity in that region). Lesions occasionally appear benign on plain radiographs and more aggressive on CT, particularly in areas such as the pelvis, where plain radiography may be suboptional. Close follow-up of such lesions, to include biopsy, may be required. CT can determine which muscle groups/anatomic compartments are affected by the tumor. This feature has important therapeutic implications (especially for soft tissue tumors rather than for bone tumors). CT can be useful in the detection of tumor recurrence following curettage or limb-salvage procedure.

The preceding paragraphs are not all-inclusive, but serve to highlight the important roles of CT in the evaluation of primary bone tumors. It is imperative to note that improperly performed biopsies (concerning the initial approach to the bone tumor) can restrict subsequent surgical options. Furthermore, because of the serious consequences of the planned surgical approach, it is probably reasonable to state that no bone tumor (especially no malignant bone tumor) should be operated on without prior CT. The cost of the CT exam and the concern for ionizing radiation resulting from the CT exam are trivial compared to the tremendous beneficial information provided by CT; such information frequently cannot be derived from other standard imaging modalities. Since the CT findings are rarely pathognomonic for a specific bone tumor,[28-30] CT must be used to augment the plain radiograph.

ACKNOWLEDGMENT

The author thanks the contributing radiologists and pathologists whose material illustrated this work, as well as the secretarial staff from the Department of Radiologic Pathology and the technical staff from the Medical Illustration Department, Armed Forces Institute of Pathology.

REFERENCES

1. Spjut HJ, Dorfman HD, Fechner RE, Ackerman LV: Tumors of bone and cartilage. Fascicle 5, Atlas of Tumor Pathology. Armed Forces Institute of Pathology, 1970, p. 29
2. Madewell JE, Ragsdale BD, Sweet DE: Radiologic and pathologic analysis of solitary bone lesions, Part I: Internal margins. Radiol Clin North Am 19 (4):715, 1981
3. Ragsdale BD, Madewell JE, Sweet DE: Radiologic and pathologic analysis of solitary bone lesions, Part II: Periosteal reactions. Radiol Clin North Am 19 (4):749, 1981
4. Sweet DE, Madewell JE, Ragsdale BD: Radiologic and pathologic analysis of solitary bone lesions, Part III: Matrix patterns. Radiol Clin North Am 19 (4):785, 1981
5. Price HI, Batnitzy S: The computed tomographic findings in benign diseases of the vertebral column. CRC Crit Rev Diagn Imaging 39–89, 1985
6. Daneman A, Martin DJ, Chan HSL: Cardiac metastases from osteosarcoma. Radiology 149:341, 1983
7. Watts FB, Jr., Zingas AP, Das L et al: Computed tomographic diagnosis of an intracardial metastasis from osterosarcoma. Radiology 151:554, 1984

8. Paling MR, Hyams DM: Computed tomography in malignant fibrous histiocytoma. Radiology 147:309, 1983
9. Karian JM, DeFilipp G, Buchheit WA et al: Vertebral osterochondroma causing spinal cord compression: case report. Neurosurgery 14:483, 1984
10. Novick GS, Pavlov H, Bullough PG: Osteochondroma of the cervical spine: report of two cases in pre-adolescent males. Skel Radiol 8:13, 1982
11. Spallone A, DiLorenzo N, Nardi P, Noletti A: Spinal osteochondroma diagnosed by computed tomography. Report of two cases and review of literature. Acta Neurochir 105, 1981
12. Kenney PJ, Gilula LA, Murphy WA: The use of computed tomography to distinguish osteo-chondroma and chondrosarcoma. Radiology 139:129, 1981
13. Norman A, Sissons HA: Radiographic hallmarks of peripheral chondrosarcoma. Radiology 151:589, 1984
14. Hudson TM, Manaster BJ: Radiology of medullary chondrosarcoma: preoperative treatment planning. Radiology 153:269, 1984
15. Adler CP, Klumper A, Wenz W: Enchondroma from a radiological and pathologic-anatomical standpoint. Radiology 134:569, 1980
16. Shapiro F: Ollier's disease. Radiology 144:969, 1982
17. Hudson TM, Hawkins IF, Jr.: Radiological evaluation of chondroblastoma. Radiology 139:1, 1981
18. Rosenthal DI, Schiller AL, Mankin HJ: Chondrosarcoma: correlation of radiological and histo-logical grade. Radiology 150:21, 1984
19. Mayes GB, Wallace S, Bernardino ME: Computed tomography of chondrosarcoma. Radiology 143:593, 1982
20. Huvos AG, Rosen G, Bretsky SS et al: Telangiectatic osteogenic sarcoma: a clinicopathologic study of 124 patients. Radiology 145:579, 1982
21. Rosenthal DI: Computed tomography in bone and soft tissue neoplasms: application and patho-logic correlation. CRC Crit Rev Diagn Imaging 18:243, 1982
22. Schumacher TM, Genant HK, Korobkin M, Bovill EG, Jr.: Computed tomography. Its use in space-occupying lesions of the musculoskeletal system. J Bone Joint Surg 60:600, 1978
23. Vaniel D, Contesso G, Couanet D et al: Computed tomography in the evaluation of 41 cases of Ewing's sarcoma. Radiology 148:888, 1983
24. Lorentzon R, Larsson SE, Boquiss L: Parosteal (juxtacortical) osteosarcoma. Radiology 136:818, 1980
25. Stovall JM, Kim A, Ventura OJ: Parosteal osteosarcoma. Radiology 146:276, 1983
26. Desantos LA, Spjut HS: Periosteal chondroma: a radiographic spectrum. Radiology 140:268, 1961
27. Bertoni F, Boriani S, Laus M: Periosteal chondrosarcoma and periosteal osteosarcoma. Radiology 146:867, 1983
28. McLeod RA, Stephens DH, Beabout JW et al: Computed tomography of the skeletal system. Semin Roentgenol 13:235, 1978
29. Yu R, Brunner DR, Rao KC: Role of computed tomography in symptomatic vertebral hemangio-mas. J Comput Assist Tomogr 8:311, 1984
30. Herrlin K, Ekelund L, Lovdahl R et al: Computed tomography in suspected osteoid osteoma of tubular bones. Radiology 148:889, 1983

3 The Role of CT in the Therapeutic Management of Soft Tissue Sarcomas

EVA S. ZINREICH
RUDOLPH ALMARAZ

Soft tissue sarcomas are uncommon lesions. In the United States approximately 4,500 new cases are diagnosed each year, accounting for 0.7 percent of all cancers.[1] Sarcomas arise largely from the mesodermal structures. Forty percent of soft tissue sarcomas occur in the lower extremity, 15 percent in the upper extremity, 30 percent in the trunk, and 15 percent in the head and neck area.[2,3] In recent years, histoanalysis and electron microscopy have contributed to more accurate pathologic classification of these soft tissue tumors.[2] The treatment of soft tissue sarcomas has changed dramatically in recent years. Once believed to have a uniformly fatal outcome, these malignancies now have improved long-term survival when a multimodality therapeutic approach is used.

The important clinical advances in the management of patients with soft tissue tumors include the development of a clinical staging system, better multidisciplinary integration, limb salvage surgery, the use of radiotherapy, and the use of chemotherapy.

STAGING

The American Joint Commission has developed a staging system based on four parameters: tumor size (T), nodal involvement (N), metastasis (M), and histologic grading of the tumor (G)[3] (Table 3-1). Histologic grade does appear to be the most useful guide to prognosis. CT contributes important information in the first three of these four categories.

CLINICAL PRESENTATION AND DIAGNOSIS

Soft tissue sarcomas most often present as asymptomatic soft tissue masses. Reliable physical signs have not been found to distinguish between benign and malignant soft tissue lesions. Often the appearance on CT scan can help

TABLE 3-1. Staging in soft tissue sarcomas

Stage I
   A: T1 N0 M0 G1
   B: T2 N0 M0 G1
Stage II
   A: T1 N0 M0 G2
   B: T2 N0 M0 G2
Stage III
   A: T1 N0 M0 G3
   B: T2 N0 M0 G3
   C: T1–2 N1 M0 G3
Stage IV
   A: T3 N0–1 M0 G1–3
   B: T1–3 N0–1 M1 G1–3

Primary tumor (T)	Nodal Involvement (N)
1 <5 cm in diameter	0 No involvement
2 >5 cm in diameter	1 Regional node involvement
3 evidence of bone invasion or invasion of major artery	

Distant Metastasis (M)	Grade (G)
0 No distant metastasis	1 Well differentiated
1 Distant metastasis present	2 Moderately well differentiated
	3 Poorly differentiated

determine the likely histologic type of a soft tissue mass. The CT scan findings of various soft tissue masses are described in Chapter 1. Only a biopsy will afford an accurate distinction. It is important to involve an experienced surgical oncologist in the early diagnostic evaluation and biopsy procedure, since the type of biopsy required is an important aspect of the overall management of the patient. Care should be taken to place the biopsy incision at a location and an orientation that do not compromise a subsequent definitive surgical excision. A large sample of tissue is often required for accurate diagnosis. Therefore, the aspiration needle technique should not play a role in the diagnosis of soft tissue tumors. Lesions smaller than 3 cm are clinically silent and only infrequently detected; for such small lesions excisional biopsy is both diagnostic and therapeutic. As a general rule, incisional biopsies are recommended for all lesions greater than 3 to 4 cm to prevent spread of malignant cells to the surrounding tissue planes. Extreme care must be used to avoid a hematoma or fascial spread. Thus, the incision should be longitudinal and not transverse. The biopsy site should be excised entirely at the time of the definitive procedure.

    Planning the surgical resection and/or radiation therapy requires a careful and detailed determination of the pattern of local spread and exact extent of the lesion, aided by certain diagnostic radiographic procedures, which should include CT scan through the affected region and the chest, and arteriography.

In most centers, xerography has been replaced by CT, although the former may still be used in the assessment of neck mases. Radiography of the soft tissue mass may delineate the soft tissue mass, and show certain structural characteristics such as tumor calcification; however, its diagnostic value has been surpassed by CT (Fig. 3-1).

Computed tomography affords the greatest accuracy in the display of tumor extension (Fig. 3-2). It is also found to be more accurate than other radiographic

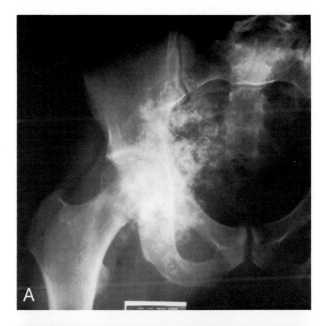

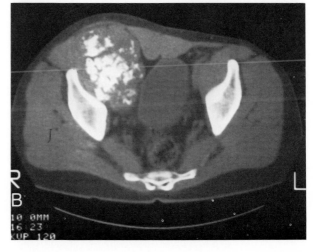

FIG. 3-1. (A) Roentgenogram of the pelvis in a 20-year-old man with chondrosarcoma involving the ilium. (B) CT scan of the pelvis shows the involved ilium with no involvement of sacroiliac joint; the patient was a candidate for hemipelvectomy.

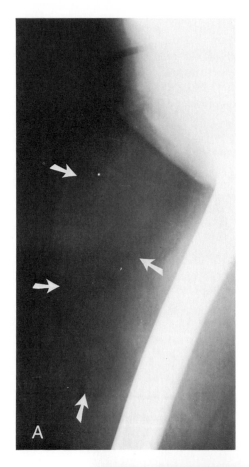

FIG. 3-2. (A) Soft tissue x-ray study of the right thigh of a patient with a large liposarcoma (arrows). (B) The extent of the lesion is best appreciated by CT scan of the right thigh (arrows).

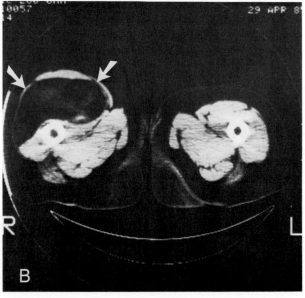

procedures in the evaluation of adjacent bony invasion as well as distant metastasis (chest CT).

If surgical resection is contemplated, arteriography is useful to determine possible involvement of major vessels in those cases in which CT examination fails to provide sufficient information. Arteriography may be necessary to determine the general status of the vascular system of an extremity in elderly patients in whom extensive arteriosclerosis might preclude successful surgery.

SURGICAL THERAPY

Originally, surgery of soft tissue sarcomas involved simple excision of gross tumor with little or no normal tissue margin. Not surprisingly, the local failure rate of this procedure was high,[4,5] approximately 80 percent. In the 1950s radical surgical procedures, such as amputation, increased local control, reducing the local failure rate to 25 to 30 percent.[6,7]

Low-grade soft tissue sarcomas require wide local excision with completely negative margins. High-grade sarcomas require radical local excisions, and must encompass the entire tumor and all tissues in the compartment in which the sarcoma is situated. This procedures involves muscle group excision, compartmental excision, and amputation, resulting in a local control rate of about 80 percent.[6,7]

Since every attempt to preserve an extremity is now advocated, surgical techniques have been devised to provide for adequate excisions while maintaining the function of the extremity. Recently, some patients with soft tissue sarcomas of the extremities have become candidates for limb-salvage procedures instead of the more mutilating amputation procedures. Improved preservation of function and substitution of salvage procedure for amputation are made possible by adjuvant radiation therapy and chemotherapy administered postoperatively. All gross tumor is removed with a minimum of 1 to 2 cm of normal tissue surrounding the sarcoma. No attempt is made to remove the entire muscle group or compartment.

Radical surgical excisions for recurrent soft tissue sarcoma or advanced primary sarcoma of the extremities often require significant soft tissue loss, thus complicating skin closures. The use of free vascular musculocutaneous flaps has provided the surgical oncologist and plastic surgeon with excellent means of providing closure of the remaining soft tissue defects in extremity surgery. The use of these flaps does not compromise the timing of administering radiation therapy because such radiation can be delivered locally through intraoperatively placed Silastic catheters in the resection bed. These catheters are loaded with radioactive materials postoperatively, allowing prompt local irradiation. This eliminates initial external irradiation of the healing free flap but provides adequate irradiation to the area at greatest risk (Fig. 3-3).

RADIATION THERAPY

The goal of radiotherapy is local control; it can be administered as primary therapy or in combination with surgery, either preoperatively or postoperatively.

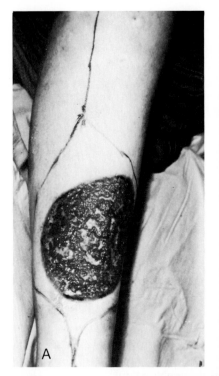

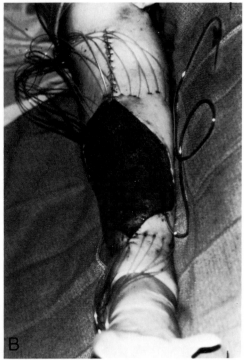

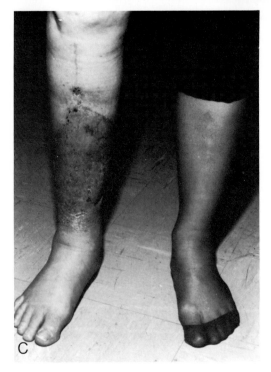

FIG. 3-3. (A) Forty-eight-year-old patient with a recurrent malignant schwannoma on the right leg after local excision of the granulated wound with positive resection margin. (B) After radical excision of the anterior compartment, plastic catheters, were left behind for later local radiation therapy using iridium[90] radioactive ribbons. A free vascular latissimus dorsi flap covers the defect and is covered by a split-thickness skin graft. (C) At the 3-month follow-up examination after resection and radiation therapy (6,000 rad), the patient has good function in the lower extremity.

Technique

In the treatment of soft tissue tumors, the first objective is to design the treatment volume and determine the tumor dose.

Treatment Volume

The radiation treatment volume encompasses all tissue suspected of being involved by tumor as well as those handled in the surgical procedure. Because of the large volume, complex treatment plans are important to exclude uninvolved tissues. In the design of the tumor volume a close collaboration between the surgeon, radiologist, and pathologist is critical. Planning is significantly aided by a preoperative CT scan to delineate accurately the exact tumor volume, or by carefully placed surgical clips at the outer margin of the surgical field or at the margins of the gross tumor.

The first step in the treatment plan is to establish a reproducible and accurate positioning of the region to be treated. For lower extremity sarcomas, immobilizing casts of the affected, or sometimes both, extremities are needed. For optimal accuracy a CT scan is obtained of the region to be treated with the immobilizing cast in position. After the proper positioning is assured, simulation films are obtained. Plaster strips are used to obtain skin contours at several levels over the area of interest. Graph paper tracings of these contours allow mapping of the anatomic landmarks and tumor volume. Computer treatment planning is then used to delineate the optimal planes for delivery of the maximum tumor dose. The anticipated dose to tumor and to adjacent normal tissues can be calculated; the ideal goal should be to minimize the dose to normal tissues (Fig. 3-4).

Tumor Dose

The initial treatment volume should be irradiated to 5,000 rads in 5 to 6 weeks. The treatment volume is then reduced to cover the size of initial tumor to a dose of 6,400 to 6,600 rads.

Definitive Radiation Therapy

Radiation is used as a definitive mode of therapy predominantly in the management of retroperitoneal sarcomas, since patients with these tumors are not candidates for definitive surgery. Patients with other sarcomas, who refuse surgery, may benefit from radiotherapy alone. Doses of 6,400 to 6,600 rads over 6 to 7 weeks are administered.

A group of 51 patients with soft tissue sarcomas were treated with radiation therapy alone at the Massachusetts General Hospital between 1970 and 1982. These patients either refused surgery or were found to have nonresectable tumors. Their 5-year survival rate was 25.1 percent and the rate of local control[9]

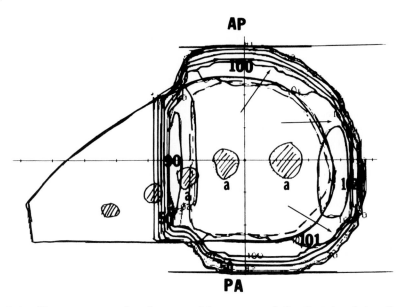

FIG. 3-4. The treatment plan for synovial sarcoma of the foot involving the first metatarsal. After resection of the tumor the patient received 6,400 rad through an anteroposterior/posteroanterior treatment portal. (Arrows show a 1-cm bolus on the skin to increase skin dose to 101 percent). a, metatarsal; AP, anterior treatment port; PA, posterior treatment port.

was 33 percent. There has been much interest in the use of radiation therapy combined with surgical resection in the treatment of sarcoma of soft tissue. A number of reports have indicated a good tumor control with the use of high-dose postoperative radiation therapy after local tumor resection.

Preoperative and Postoperative Radiotherapy

More recently, there has been some resumed interest and research in the use of primary preoperative radiation therapy, with excellent local control reported, especially in the treatment of advanced soft tissue tumors.

Preoperative radiation therapy consists of the delivery of 5,000 rads prior to en bloc resection of the soft tissue sarcoma. Preoperative radiation therapy was used in the treatment of 36 patients with soft tissue sarcomas at the Massachusetts General Hospital.[10] The dose of 5,000 to 6,000 rads over 6 weeks was followed by a conservative resection 3 weeks later, followed by a booster dose, intraoperatively or postoperatively (1,000 to 1,500 rad). Local control was excellent in 31 of 33 patients over a follow-up interval of 3 months to 8 years. Three of the 33 patients could not undergo surgery and had further radiotherapy. Tumor in two of these three patients recurred locally. Wound healing was delayed in 6 of the 30 patients.[10] A recent review comparing 60 patients who received primary preoperative radiation therapy and 110 who received primary postoperative radiation therapy revealed similar local control with both procedures. Patients with large soft tissue sarcomas seemed to have improved local control when preoperative radiation therapy was used.[11]

The advantages of preoperative irradiation include

1.   The treatment volume is designed to include only those tissues known to be involved by tumor (based on the CT scan) and those tissues suspected of microscopic extension. In contrast, postoperative radiotherapy tumor volume must cover not only what is described above but also all tissue handled during the surgical procedure, thus making the treatment volume larger than preoperatively.

2.   Preoperative radiation is expected to inactivate the tumor cells and consequently decrease the chances for viable tumor cells to metastasize during surgical manipulation.

3.   If the tumor mass regresses considerably during preoperative radiotherapy, this will facilitate conservative resection; thus a previously unresectable tumor may become resectable.

4.   There is no delay in starting radiotherapy.

5.   There is seldom a problem with wound healing.

The disadvantages of preoperative therapy include

1.   Delay of surgery (7 to 9 weeks).

2.   Continued and likely increased patient anxiety due to prolongation of the tumor removal.

3.   The whole tumor specimen is not available for tissue diagnosis at the initial therapy.

Further investigation of primary preoperative treatment is in progress, but at this time most centers prefer to treat soft tissue sarcomas postoperatively with a dose of 6,400 to 6,600 rads over 6 weeks. The extent of surgery varies from a gross resection to compartmental resection. Radiation therapy is planned 2 weeks postoperatively as described above. The local control achieved with postoperative radiotherapy is 80 percent, with a survival rate of 70 percent at 5 years, shown[11-13] in Table 3-2.

TABLE 3-2.   Results of postoperative radiation therapy in the treatment of soft tissue sarcomas

Institution	No. of patients	Survival (%) 2 years	Survival (%) 5 years	Local Control (%)
Massachusetts General Hospital[11]	110		69	87.9
M. D. Anderson Hospital[12]	300	74	61.3	78.7
University of California[13]	47		73	90

CHEMOTHERAPY

Soft tissue sarcomas are characterized by aggressive soft tissue invasion and early metastases to the lungs. Several chemotherapeutic agents are effective in achieving objective, although temporary, regression of metastasis.

Currently, the best agents are doxorubicin (Adriamycin), cyclophosphamide (Cytoxan); dimethyl sulfoxide, triazeno-imidazole-carboxamide (DTIC); vincristine, methotrexate, and cis-platinum.

Since 1975 the National Cancer Institute has studied the role of adjuvant chemotherapy in a randomized study of 65 patients with high-grade soft tissue sarcomas. The chemotherapeutic regimen included doxorubicin (50 mg/m², escalated by 10 mg/m² increments to a maximum of 70 mg/m²), cyclophosphamide (500 mg/m², escalated by 100 mg/m² increments to a maximum of 700 mg/m²), and methotrexate (50 mg/kg to a maximum of 250 mg/kg).[14]

In this group, local therapy included either surgical amputation or wide local resection combined with radiation therapy. Thirty-seven patients received chemotherapy, starting in the immediate postoperative period. Ninety-two percent of the patients receiving chemotherapy were disease-free at 3 years, compared with 60 percent in the nonchemotherapy group. Local failure was absent in the former group, with only two local failures occurring in the latter group.[14]

Rosenberg, treating 37 patients with sarcoma involving the trunk, head, neck, and breast (excluding retroperitoneal tumors), added doxorubicin and cyclophosphamide and methotrexate to the conventional surgical and/or radiation therapy and showed improvement in disease-free survival. Three-year actuarial survival rate was 90 percent in the chemotherapy group and 46 percent in the group receiving only conventional surgery and/or radiation therapy.[15]

The value of chemotherapy in the treatment of high-grade soft tissue sarcomas remains somewhat controversial. Recent studies indicate that chemotherapy improves disease-free survival and overall survival.

For metastatic soft tissue sarcomas, chemotherapy can produce a partial remission that is usually of relatively short duration. Complete remission occurs in only 10 to 15 percent of patients.

RETROPERITONEAL SARCOMAS

Approximately 10 to 20 percent of all soft tissue sarcomas are retroperitoneal in origin. Liposarcoma, leiomyosarcoma, and fibrosarcoma are the most common cell types.

The predominant clinical presentation at time of diagnosis is a large tumor mass and pain. Radiographic studies may show extrinsic mass effect in barium contrast studies and displacement of the ureters on intravenous pyelography. Angiography is nonspecific, showing a variety of vascular changes none of which are characteristic for a particular histologic picture. It is predominantly used to outline the major vascular channels in relation to the tumor mass preoperatively.

Computed axial tomography is the most useful radiologic test of patients with retroperitoneal sarcoma. The study affords an accurate display of size, consistency, and radiologic relationships between tumor and contiguous retroperitoneal structures (Fig. 3-5). Postresection follow-up scans are vital in the

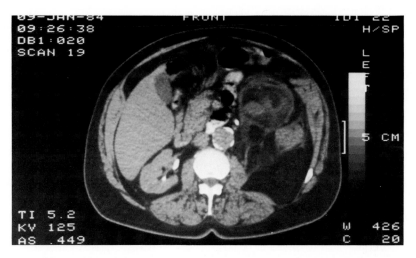

FIG. 3-5. CT scan of the abdomen in a 70-year-old man with a large liposarcoma of the retroperitoneum, who underwent complete resection and postoperative radiotherapy.

evaluation for possible tumor recurrence. Treatment of choice in retroperitoneal sarcomas has been surgical resection, with 0 to 21 percent of patients surviving and free of disease at 5 years. Twenty percent of the patients may require partial colon resection and 25 percent may require nephrectomy. Essential surgical technique includes a long vertical incision or transverse abdominal incision for adequate exposure and en bloc excision of involved adjacent organs. The dissection should extend well outside of the tumor pseudocapsule. In some patients, proximity of vital structures may preclude resection with wide, uninvolved margins. Even if all gross disease cannot be removed, every effort should be made to resect as much as possible to reduce the bulk of residual disease.

Adjuvant therapy in retroperitoneal sarcomas includes pre- or postoperative radiotherapy. Table 3-3 reviews the result of the therapy in retroperitoneal sarcoma.[16,17]

TABLE 3-3. Survival of patients with retroperitoneal sarcoma

Institution	No. of patients	Therapy	5-Year Survival (%)	Local Control (%)
Massachusetts General Hospital[16]	17	Curative therapy 5,000–6,900 rad	54	54
Memorial Hospital[17]	128	Incomplete excision	3	
	77	Complete excision	40	33
			22: No evidence of disease	

The value of adjuvant chemotherapy is being evaluated by a number of investigators. Rosenberg et al. used adjuvant chemotherapy with Adriamycin and Cytoxan in a randomized study of soft tissue sarcomas at all sites. While results in those with retroperitoneal sarcoma were unchanged, there was improved survival in patients with sarcomas of the extremities.

DESMOID TUMORS

Desmoid tumors are rare, slow-growing, benign fibrous neoplasms that arise from fascial sheaths and muscoloaponeurotic structures. They were initially described in the abdominal wall of postpartum women. It is now recognized that these tumors may arise in any anatomic location (Fig. 3-6).

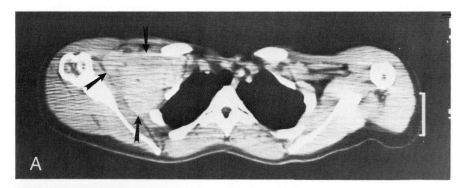

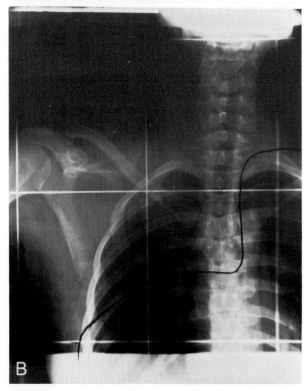

FIG. 3-6. (A) CT scan of a desmoid tumor of the right shoulder was performed in a 23-year-old woman for planning of definitive radiation therapy (arrows). (B) The radiation therapy port, including the mass with generous margins.

Initial treatment currently consists of wide local surgical resection; however, the infiltrative behavior of this tumor results in a high (25 to 75 percent) incidence of local recurrence following curative surgery.

Radiation therapy may offer an excellent means of local control for tumors found to be unresectable due to their location or extension. Leibel, using 5,000 to 5,500 rads over 5 to 6 weeks, reported a 5-year relapse-free survival of 72 percent. The regression of these tumors following radiotherapy is slow, requiring up to 2 years.[18]

Postoperative radiotherapy may prevent local recurrence when the tumor is found at or close to the surgical margins.

SUMMARY

The accepted treatment of primary soft tissue sarcomas has evolved rapidly during the last few decades.

A multidisciplinary approach, better preoperative localization, and characterization using CT, less-radical surgery, and radiation therapy and/or chemotherapy permitted the formulation of reasonable limb-saving procedures with good local control (Fig. 3-7).

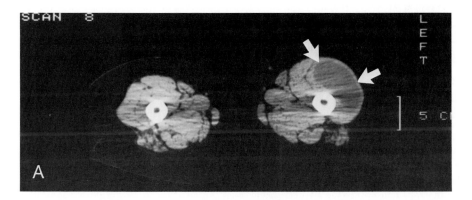

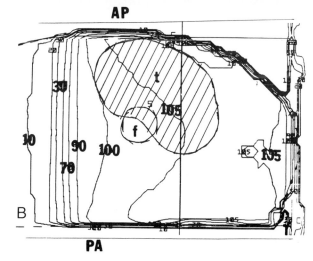

FIG. 3-7. A 34-year-old woman with grade 3 liposarcoma of the thigh was treated with compartmental resection followed by postoperative radiation therapy and chemotherapy. (A) CT scan of the thigh with mass in lateral compartment (arrows). (B) Treatment plan using an anterior and a posterior beam to cover the tumor volume 100 percent. AP, anterior beam; PA, posterior beam.

The success of this therapeutic approach depends on close collaboration of the surgeon, radiologist, pathologist, and radiation oncologist.

REFERENCES

1. Sieverberg E: Cancer statistics. Ca 31:13, 1981
2. Linberg RD, Martin RG, Romsdahl MM: Surgery and postoperative radiotherapy in the treatment of soft tissue sarcomas in adults. Am J Roentgenol 123:123, 1975
3. Russel WO, Cohen J, Enzinger FM et al: A clinical and pathological staging system for soft tissue sarcomas. Cancer 40:1562, 1977
4. Martin RG, Buttler JJ, Albores Saavedra J: Soft Tissue Tumors: Surgical Treatment and Results for Tumors of Bone and Soft Tissues. Year Book, Chicago, 1965
5. Cantin J, McNeer GP, Chu FC et al: The problem of local recurrence after treatment of soft tissue sarcoma. Ann Surg 168:47, 1968
6. Simon MA, Enneking WF: The management of soft tissue sarcomas of the extremities. J Bone Joint Surg 58A:317, 1976
7. Shiu MH, Castro EB, Hajdu SI et al: Surgical treatment of 297 soft tissue sarcomas of lower extremity. Ann Surg 182:597, 1975
8. Tepper J, Rosenberg AS, Glatstein E: Radiation therapy technique in soft tissue sarcomas of the extremity—policies of treatment at the National Cancer Institutes. Int J Radiation Oncol 8:263, 1982
9. Tepper EJ, Suit HD: Radiation therapy alone for sarcoma of soft tissue. Cancer 56:475, 1985
10. Suit HD, Proppe KH, Mankin JH, Wood WC: Preoperative radiation therapy for sarcoma of soft tissue. Cancer 47:2269, 1981
11. Suit HD, Mankin HJ, Wood WC et al: Preoperative, intraoperative, postoperative radiation in the treatment of primary soft tissue sarcoma. Cancer 55:2659, 1985
12. Lindbert RD, Martin RG, Romsdahl MM et al: Conservative surgery and postoperative radiotherapy in 300 adults with soft-tissue sarcomas. Cancer 47:2391, 1981
13. Leibel SA, Tranbaugh RF, Wara WM et al: Soft tissue sarcomas of the extremities—survival and patterns of failure with conservative surgery and postoperative irradiation compared to surgery alone. Cancer 50:1076, 1982
14. Rosenberg SA, Tepper J, Glatstein E et al: Prospective randomized evaluation of adjuvant chemotherapy in adults with soft tissue sarcomas of the extremities. Cancer 52:424, 1983
15. Glenn J, Kinsella T, Glatstein E et al: A randomized, prospective trial of adjuvant chemotherapy in adults with soft tissue sarcomas of the head and neck, breast, and trunk. Cancer 55:1206, 1985
16. Tepper JE, Suit HD, Wood WC et al: Radiation therapy of retroperitoneal soft tissue sarcomas. Int J Radiation Oncol 10:825, 1982
17. Cody HS, Turnbull AD, Fortner JG et al: The continuing challenge of retroperitoneal sarcomas. Cancer 47:2147, 1981
18. Leibel SA, Wara WM, Hill DR et al: Desmoid tumors: local control and patterns of relapse following radiation therapy. Int J Radiation Oncol 9:1167, 1983

4 Assessment of Musculoskeletal Inflammation

DONNA MAGID
ELLIOT K. FISHMAN

Inflammatory disease of the musculoskeletal system is a potentially life-threatening problem that frequently presents as a diagnostic dilemma. While the presence of inflammatory disease may be announced by clinical and laboratory findings and roughly localized by physical examination, conclusive characterization of the lesion, localization to tissue compartment, and exclusion of other diagnostic possibilities can remain elusive.

The plain roentgenographic detection of inflammatory disease is markedly limited in the evaluation of the soft tissue component of inflammatory disease. While there may be subtle clues, such as distortion of fat/tissue planes or detection of gas within soft tissue, the negative plain film examination does not rule out significant, often extensive, disease. Plain film cannot readily localize an inflammatory lesion to compartment (subcutaneous tissue, muscle, bone, joint), nor accurately map the boundaries of such a lesion. Early detection or confirmation of lesions is precluded by the insensitivity of plain film to soft tissue changes, and by the biologic time frame required for radiographically detectable alterations in bone.[1]

Computed tomography addresses most, if not all, of these issues. Its superior sensitivity to minor differences in tissue attenuation can be augmented by comparison to the (normal) contralateral part and by manipulation of window center and width. Localization to tissue compartment is simplified; for example, it can differentiate superficial primary cellulitis from that secondary to deeper disease of muscle or bone. Abscess or fluid collections can be detected and drained with best access confirmed by CT. Even small, deep gas collections, which are potential surgical emergencies, can be localized and characterized.

Techniques parallel those used for other musculoskeletal problems. Fastidious positioning and patient instruction ensure bilateral symmetry for comparison. Eight-millimeter collimation at 8-mm intervals is used routinely, with 4 mm by 4 mm used for smaller parts (e.g., joint space, tarsal area). Higher scanning techniques such as 5.2 sec., 450 MAS, 120 kVp (Siemans DR-3 scanner) are used to help accentuate subtle differences in tissue attenuation. Multiplanar reconstruction is not routinely performed. Intravenous enhancement increases the density distinction between normal (enhancing) soft tissue and abnormal areas of inflammation. Soft tissue abscess may show some rim enhancement. While contrast amplifies the demarcation between normal and abnormal, definite distinction among inflammatory, neoplastic, and traumatic soft tissue abnormalities may not be possible (although most neoplasms are more vascular). With long-standing inflammatory disease, some neovascularization or enhanced vascular supply may be demonstrated. As with all studies, all images are reviewed and filmed at bone and soft tissue windows, with adjustment of windows as necessary to emphasize subtle findings.

CELLULITIS

While cellulitis is a clinical diagnosis, it may be difficult to assess the depth to which inflammation penetrates. Cellulitis may be a superficial inflammation in isolation, a superficial inflammation penetrating the deeper layers, or may be secondary to a deeper or more chronic process surfacing. Acute superficial cellulitis is a subcutaneous inflammation usually lacking a necrotic or suppurative response, but can lead to tissue necrosis and abscess formation. Such an infection will spread along fascial planes and may involve the lymphatic drainage. Cellulitis may also form in reaction to underlying inflammation such as osteomyelitis, or to superinfection of chronic cutaneous ulcers. Prompt and appropriate management is essential since primary cellulitis can progress to abscess or myonecrosis, while secondary cellulitis may represent just one aspect of a serious underlying process.

Conventional radiographic signs can be subtle and may not cause clinical symptoms for days or even weeks. Soft tissue planes are poorly depicted on plain film, and it may difficult to assess the depth and extent of each compartment's involvement. Plain films are frequently requested in patients with cellulitis or infected decubiti ulcers to rule out underlying osteomyelitis, but the lag between symptoms and radiographic signs (10 to 21 days) is a significant obstacle to appropriate management.[1] Radionuclide bone scan followed by gallium citrate scan may help to identify, and to a lesser extent, localize infection and frequently can be diagnostic within 24 hours of the onset of symptoms.[2] However, such studies fail to provide adequate definition of the anatomy of involvement.

In cellulitis, infiltration predominates over mass effect. Computed tomography will demonstrate minimal swelling as a focal or diffuse expansion of normal features, with the contralateral side helping in the appreciation of subtle alterations of size, contour, or texture. Cellulitis produces inflammation and edema of the subcutaneous fat, raising its CT attenuation values (normal −90 to −120 Hounsfield units (HU) and obliterating the sharp distinction from underlying muscle and soft tissue. With intravenous contrast, some hypervascularity may be appreciated as asymmetrical enhancement in comparison to more normal tissue. CT may confirm the superficial nature of the lesion, with only minimal local deeper reaction, or may show tissue necrosis or abscess formation. The accumulation of previously undetected pus is an indication for drainage, with CT documenting both the need and the best interventional approach. Very local and well-defined fluid collections may be adequately drained via CT or sonographic guided puncture, while loculated or more complex collections may require surgical debridement for adequate drainage. In those patients with cellulitis secondary to infection of decubitus ulcers, burns, or soft tissue defects from trauma or surgery, CT may help in planning grafting or other reconstructive procedures.

Since cellulitis juxtaposed to bone can provoke a reactive periostitis, CT distinction of a primary soft tissue process from one secondary to osteomyelitis may not be possible. However, the cortex remains essentially unchanged in the former, while with osteomyelitis there may be slight alterations in cortical medullary densities (see below).

LYMPHEDEMA

Conventional radiography is limited in the assessment of soft tissue swelling and edema of the extremities. Such swelling may be secondary to trauma, systemic disease such as anasarca or chronic congestive heart failure, venous insufficiency, lymphatic disease, or soft tissue infection or inflammation.

Lymphedema may be primary, with abnormal lymphatic anatomy and drainage, or secondary to any acquired process resulting in lymphatic obstruction or insult (*Wucheria bancrofti* infestation, chronic infection with lymphatic thrombosis, burns, radiation therapy, surgery, trauma, malignant disease, or abscess). The characteristic painless swelling of lymphedema is rubbery and nonpitting. If the condition becomes chronic, the skin and subcutaneous tissues begin to fibrose and thicken, with late papillary changes in the skin (lymphostatic verrucosis). The protein-rich fluid is a good culture medium and complications include recurrent beta-hemolytic streptococcal cellulitis and lymphangitis. Rarely (and most commonly with lymphedema secondary to mastectomy) lymphangiosarcoma is seen complicating chronic lymphedema.[3]

Lymphangiography is a technically difficult procedure with a significant rate of complications. Furthermore, it gives little or no information about other soft tissues, and takes several days to complete. Distal obstruction compromises visualization of more proximal structures. Computed tomography is a rapid and relatively noninvasive means of investigating the patient with chronic swelling and edema and in investigating problems associated with any of the processes in the differential diagnosis of lymphedema. Previously described CT findings include increasing thickness of the subcutaneous compartment, usually in conjunction with skin thickening. The subcutaneous tissue frequently has a nonenhancing "honeycomb" appearance, with apparent fatty pockets distributed through fluid and/or fibrous tissue. The subfascial compartment remains normal.[4,5] Since the subcutaneous thickening represents fibrous replacement, these changes are of soft tissue (20 HU) density (Fig. 4-1). While chronic

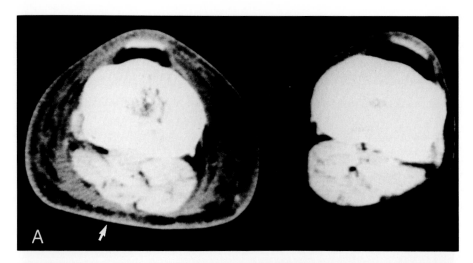

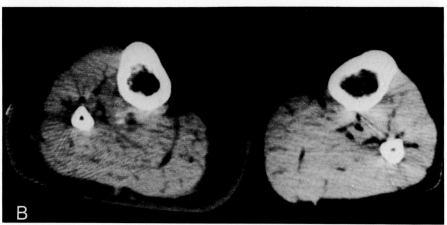

FIG. 4-1. (A) Lymphedema in a 31-year-old man with painless swelling of the right leg. At the level of the patella, a noncontrast CT (WW 221, WC 21) shows diffuse enlargement of the subcutaneous compartment, criss-crossed by soft-tissue density honeycombing, and marked skin thickening (arrow). The muscle compartment remains essentially symmetrical with the normal left leg. (B) At the level of the proximal tibial shaft, narrowed windows (WW 164, WC −8) accentuate the subcutaneous honeycombing and skin thickening.

venous disease may produce similar skin and subcutaneous alterations, it lacks this honeycomb appearance, and may demonstrate subfascial abnormalities as well. Lymphedema may be well-localized or, with more central (e.g., pelvic) primary insults, bilateral, although asymmetrical; CT will study both sides simultaneously. The primary cause (abscess, pelvic neoplasm and/or adenopathy, or postoperative changes) usually can also be characterized by CT.

MYONECROSIS

Myonecrosis most commonly is associated with posttraumatic or postsurgical contamination, classically with *Clostridium perfringens,* but occasionally with nonclostridial agents. Extensive muscular damage, compromised arterial supply and tissue anoxia, and foreign matter contamination all favor myonecrosis. The destructive capacity of clostridia, an extremely invasive agent, probably stems from the production of various exotoxins, although enzymatic inhibition and acidosis may also contribute.[3,6] Primary myonecrosis progresses aggressively from the onset of acute pain and is considered a surgical emergency. Myonecrosis secondary to clostridial cellulitis may be less toxic, and is a rare complication of such a cellulitis, since cellulitis does not commonly penetrate. A form of myonecrosis seen in comatose or drug abusing patients with prolonged immobility is believed to result from neurovascular compromise and muscle compartment syndrome with similar local and systemic effects.[7] In the patient with clinical or radiologic findings that suggest soft tissue gas, CT will help to rule out gas accumulation due to necrotizing fascitis, a streptococcal

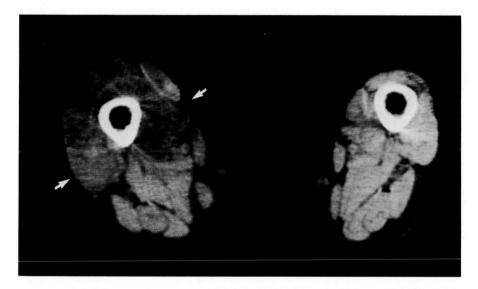

FIG. 4-2. Myonecrosis in a 37-year-old diabetic woman with minor trauma to right thigh (the side used for insulin injections) 10 days prior to CT. She was admitted for acute pain, swelling, and fever. Noncontrast CT showed diffuse swelling of the right thigh, with some inflammatory changes in the subcutaneous compartment similar to Figure 4-1. However, there is little if any skin thickening, and the most striking change is a well-demarcated engorgement and edema of the muscles of the anterior compartment (vastus lateralis, intermedius, and medialis) (arrows) with sparing of the medial and posterior compartments. Surgically proven myonecrosis was documented, with cultures negative for bacterial, viral, or fungal infection, presumably due to diabetic vascular compromise combined with acute and chronic trauma.

infection of the fascia and subcutaneous tissue, or to crepitant cellulitis alone, which may cause penetration of gas into subcutaneous or fascial planes, but usually spares muscle. In the patient with crepitant or clostridial cellulitis, CT promptly determines the presence or, more commonly, the absence of underlying muscular involvement.[8]

True muscular necrosis is seen as an area of lower tissue attenuation (20 to 40 HU) in a swollen or distorted muscle (Fig. 4-2). Accumulated gas may be finely divided and distributed between muscle fibers in a "feathery" or delicate pattern.[9] Early compromise of vascular supply produces a minimally or nonenhancing lesion that may be well demarcated.[7] In the patient with mechanical myonecrosis (e.g., drug abuse with prolonged unconsciousness), CT may help rule out deep venous thrombosis (more diffuse swelling, higher tissue attenuation, and persisting enhancement), or hematoma (initially hyperdense, resolving into a hypodense lesion with or without rim enhancement).[10] CT maps the area of involvement, which may influence surgical decisions regarding compartmental release, amputation, or other procedure.

OSTEOMYELITIS

Osteomyelitis depends on and results from an interaction of both pathogenic and host factors. Its clinical and radiographic manifestations can vary, confusing the clinical picture and delaying the early diagnosis and treatment that are essential to its satisfactory eradication.

Agents may be introduced hematogenously, tending to result in a characteristic distribution determined by vascular supply, via extension from a contiguous site, or by direct innoculation via penetrating trauma or surgery. Host susceptibility may be enhanced by systemic factors (e.g., immunosuppression, diabetes, or sickle cell anemia) or local conditions (vascular compromise or tissue necrosis) favoring successful colonization by any route.[11]

Hematogenous or primary osteomyelitis illustrates the basic sequence of events seen in bone infection. The vascular anatomy of the metaphyseal medullary cavity favors the propagation of blood-borne pathogens. The bone is functionally a closed space, and as exudate and edema expand within the rigid bone confines, intramedullary tissue pressure rises. This produces venous stasis and eventually tissue necrosis, further fostering the infection. Infection spreads along the medullary cavity and into the cortical canals. The local alterations in pH and the accumulated bacterial products, neutrophilic enzymes, and debris act as osteoclastic stimulating factors. The osteoclasts increase both in size and number.[12] Subtle cortical fissuring may be produced as the haversian and Volkmann's canals are expanded by these stimulated osteoclasts.[13] With rising tissue pressure, the cortex may decompress into the subperiosteal zone, stimulating diaphyseal periosteal reaction. Osteoclasts and proteolytic enzymes begin to resorb dead bone at its interface with viable bone and granulation tissue, with cancellous bone being more readily resorbed (2 to 3 weeks) than cortex (2 to 24 weeks).[14] New bone will be laid down along the remaining scaffolding and by the stimulated periosteum, with full mineralization of matrix taking approximately 10 days.[1]

In a process where early identification and aggressive treatment are imperative, conventional radiographic signs are notoriously slow to develop. The earliest plain film indication may be soft tissue edema and swelling. The initial osseous manifestation—local demineralization and osteoporosis—may require 7 to 14 days to advance sufficiently (30 to 50 percent mineral loss) to be appreciated on plain film.[1] Fine cortical fissures representing the marked expansion of the cortical canals may precede decompression into the subperiosteal space.[13] Subperiosteal new bone mineralization lags behind the lytic processes, prolonging to approximately 3 to 6 weeks the gap between the onset of infection and radiographic evidence of new bone formation.

Computed tomography provides an elegant analysis of tissue interfaces, anatomy, and density, separating and assessing the compartmentalized (soft tissue, medullary cavity, cortex, and periosteum) changes of osteomyelitis (Figs. 4-3, 4-4) and facilitating earlier diagnosis and treatment. Normal diaphyseal marrow measures fat density (-100 to -120 HU).[15,16] The gradual interdigitation of cancellous bone and marrow in the metaphyseal medullary cavity leads to a gradual rise from negative medullary attenuation to the positive CT attenuation of the subepiphyseal cancellous bone.[16] With hematogenous infection, the earliest change is congestion and/or vascular edema in the medullary cavity, thus elevating the local radiographic attenuation. While other conditions (e.g., thalassemia, tumor infiltration, sickle cell disease, and healing fracture) can elevate marrow density, the changes are often extensive and (except with tumor or fracture) may be bilaterally symmetrical.[15] Occasionally intramedullary gas may be detected, suggesting the presence of gas-forming bacterial infection.[17] Intramedullary fat/fluid levels have also been described.[18] Overlying soft tissue swelling may be seen as alterations in density and contour of adjacent soft tissue planes, with the availability of the contralateral normal side for comparison increasing the sensitivity to subtle changes. Alterations in cortical texture reflecting the expansion of the horizontal (Volkmann's) and vertical (haversian) canals, and subsequent cortical destruction, can be detected on CT long before they are visible on plain films. Focal cortical disruptions and abscesses may be noted and mapped for diagnostic biopsy (Figs. 4-3B, 4-5). More diffuse cortical thickening and irregularity, both periosteal and endosteal, may be seen with infection and reaction. Periosteal elevation and reaction can be seen before it becomes distinct on plain film, with CT's superior spatial resolution and sensitivity to small differences in density. This also allows earlier recognition of new bone formation with the attenuation of nonossified osteoid (20 to 40 HU) gradually rising as normal bone mineral accumulates.

Computed tomography evaluates long-standing or recurrent osteomyelitis, providing significant clinical guidance in persisting disease (Figs. 4-5 to 4-8). With the chronic condition, abscesses may form in overlying soft tissue, medullary cavity, or destroyed cortex (Figs. 4-5B, 4-6A, 4-7B). Subcutaneous sinus tracts may drain such cortical collections (Fig. 4-8A), and can transmit or shelter

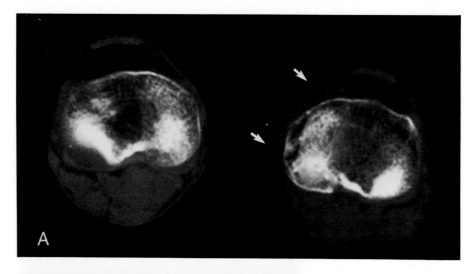

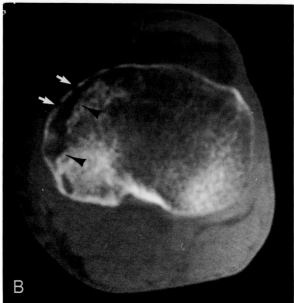

FIG. 4-3. (A) Unenhanced CT scan of a 34-year-old black man with biopsy-proven osteomyelitis of the right distal femur shows moderate medial soft tissue swelling and edema (arrows) compared to the normal left side. Irregular subcortical erosion can be seen in the medial aspect of the metaphysis. (B) Expand mode scan of (A) at wider bone window, better demonstrates subcortical destruction (black arrows) in the distal metaphysis and defines focal cortical disruptions (white arrows). This site was chosen for diagnostic biopsy.

the agents of infection. Similarly to sequestra, such tracts are relatively protected from circulating antibiotics. Occasionally, foreign bodies may be identified. Bony sequestra may be small and masked by adjacent reactive sclerosis, but can harbor active infection and should be removed (Fig. 4-8B). Soft tissue abscesses appear as lower-density collections within the soft tissue. The periphery of an abscess may enhance with intravenous contrast. Complications such as pathologic fracture, joint destruction, or extension of infection can also be confirmed (Figs. 4-5C, 4-6). CT documents the need for and facilitates planning

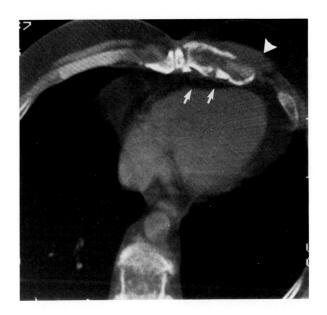

FIG. 4-4. Fifty-eight-year-old man with previous sterotomy for chest surgery, with biopsy-proven osteomyelitis. The left half of the sternum is expanded with irregular cortex. There is minimal prominence of overlying muscle (arrowhead) in comparison to the normal right chest wall. Normal epicardial fat attenuation dorsal to involved bone (arrows) is evidence against mediastinal extension.

of diagnostic needle biopsy, therapeutic aspiration, and drainage or surgical debridement. The true extent of medullary, cortical, and soft tissue involvement will be clarified, as in more acute cases.[19,20]

Two areas where CT has proven particularly helpful in the detection and characterization of osteomyelitis are the spine and the sacroiliac (SI) joint. Both structures are complicated collections of bony contours and articular surfaces best appreciated by the cross-sectional orientation of transaxial CT, augmented by multiplanar reconstructions where indicated.

Both regions have special anatomic considerations, but serve to illustrate some of the applications and advantages of CT in inflammatory disease.

Spine

Infectious spondylitis is a relatively rare disease, accounting for 2 to 4 percent of all cases of osteomyelitis; but an increasing incidence has been noted over the last 10 to 15 years. This increase is partially attributed to the prolonged survival of the immunocompromised host, widespread intravenous drug abuse, more aggressive instrumentation of the gastrointestinal and genitourinary tracts, and the trend toward use of long-term indwelling catheters.[21-23] Antegrade (arterial) or retrograde (Batson's venous plexus) hematogenous spread remains the most common route of infection, with a smaller percentage of cases resulting from direct inoculation (e.g., penetrating trauma or surgical instrumentation) or contiguous spread (e.g., intraabdominal or pelvic abscess). With hematogenous transmission, agents may lodge anywhere, including the posterior elements, epidural space, or paravertebral soft tissues, but tend to involve the

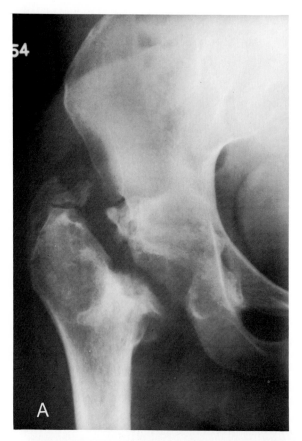

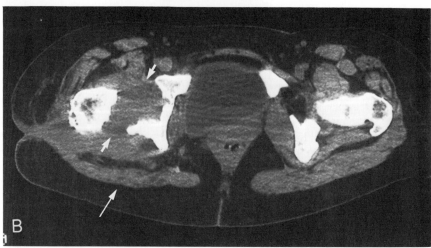

FIG. 4-5. (A) Thirty-six-year-old woman with history of systemic lupus erythematosus and previous girdlestone procedure for infected arthroplasty, followed to apparent resolution. She had new complaints of hip pain and swelling with acute exacerbation just prior to admission. Plain film is compatible with surgical deformity and findings were apparently unchanged from previous exams. (B) Noncontrast CT through the level of the left greater trochanter. Soft tissue windows show a low-attenuation abscess collection (arrows) between the right acetabulum and a minimally displaced proximal femoral remnant. There is probably involvement of muscle groups surrounding the hip although postoperative distortion complicates this analysis. Note atrophy of the gluteus maximus (arrow) compared to the normal left.

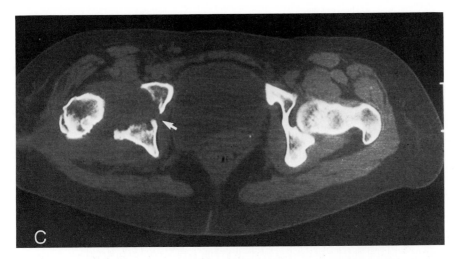

FIG. 4-5. (*Continued*) (C) CT scan just caudal to (B), bone windows. A pathologic fracture of the cotyloid fossa of the acetabulum medial wall is seen (arrow). Irregularity of the posterior acetabular surface and of the proximal femoral cortex were proven to be osteomyelitis superimposed on postoperative deformities, and probably secondary to septic arthritis.

subchondral bone near the anterior aspect of the end plate. A successfully established infection can expand from here into the disc or the anterior longitudinal ligament, while findings on conventional radiography remain unremarkable. Over the first 3 weeks of active infection, early plain film findings will include narrowing or irregularity of the disc space, loss of definition of adjacent subchondral bone, and, occasionally, widening of paravertebral soft tissue contours. Involvement of the disc allows spread to the adjacent vertebral body. In time, reactive sclerosis and/or paravertebral masses may be seen, with increasing destruction and erosion of bone (Fig. 4-9). Inflammatory masses, bony fragments, or decompressing pus may encroach upon the spinal canal, constituting a potentially life-threatening complication[22] (Fig. 4-10).

Computed tomography visualizes paravertebral soft tissues, bony structures, disc space, and spinal canal without the impediment of superimposition and allows early appreciation of subtle alterations in density or contour. The cortical margin of the vertebral body end-plate and the underlying cancellous bone usually are well defined even with routine scanning parameters; trabecular alteration and erosion will be detected far earlier than corresponding plain film findings. Additional high-resolution images may better define trabecular texture and alteration. While the disc space alterations may be more difficult to appreciate on conventional transaxial CT (where they parallel the plane of scanning), sagittal reconstructions clarify the anatomy of this area[24,25] (Fig. 4-7C). Inflammatory soft tissue masses can be distinguished from contiguous normal soft tissue by narrowing the windows, thereby accentuating the subtle attenuation differences and boundaries. Paravertebral abscesses tend to be of

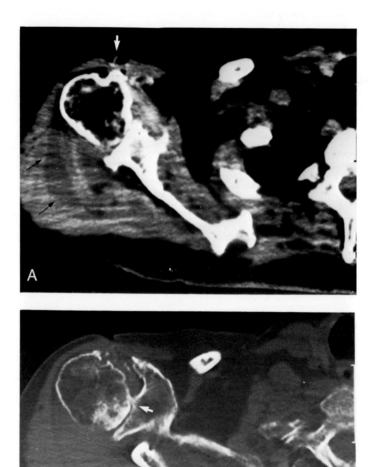

FIG. 4-6. (A) CT performed for increasing pain and fever in a 46-year-old man on steroids for glioma, with proven staphlococcal osteomyelitis, right shoulder. Soft tissue windows (WW 172, WC 21) show anterior skin and tissue deformity (white arrow) from previous abscess drainage. A large, locular, low-attenuation collection (black arrows) represents a previously unsuspected posterior abscess, which was drained. (B) This patient also complained of painful loss of range of motion with a "grating sensation." Bone windows reveal marked narrowing of the glerohumeral joint, with impingement anteriorly (arrow) that accounts for these symptoms. Subchondral sclerosis is seen below the articular surface of the humeral head, with diffuse irregularity of the humeral head.

lower attenuation than the surrounding soft tissue, and may demonstrate rim enhancement when intravenous contrast is used. Gas collections may be identified with certain pyogenic infections. Loculi can be identified and localized where therapeutic or diagnostic drainage is planned.

Computed tomography may also help identify the primary infectious source. It will also identify potentially dangerous epidural masses that may be acute

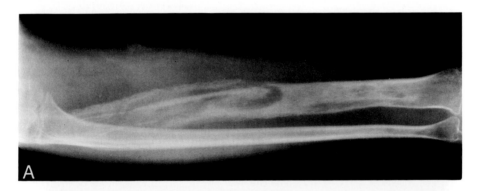

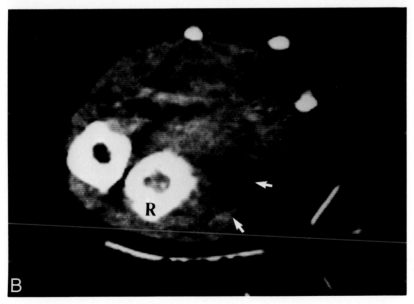

FIG. 4-7. (A) Results in a 17-year-old black girl with sickle cell anemia and complaint of 5-weeks' pain and swelling of the right forearm, sharply increasing following minor trauma just prior to admission. Plain film shows diffuse, mottled, sclerotic, and lytic changes with extensive periosteal reaction along the radial cortex. (B) CT scan with intravenous contrast, proximal forearm. Muscle windows show diffuse soft tissue swelling with obliteration of muscle planes, with a 2 × 2 cm low-attenuation collection (arrows) lateral to the radius (R), which proved to be an abscess. The attenuation of the radial medullary cavity is higher than that of the ulna.

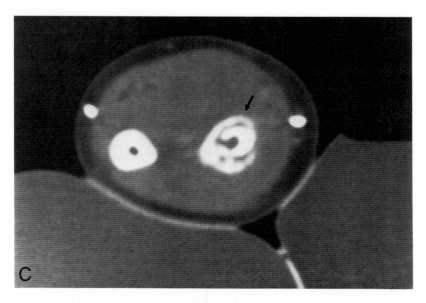

C

FIG. 4-7. (*Continued*)   (C) CT scan of the mid-forearm with intravenous contrast. Bone windows demonstrate an involucrum (arrow) cloaking the radial cortex. The focal cortical discontinuity corresponds to the level of a pathologic fracture poorly defined on plain roentgenogram.

accumulations of frank pus early in the course of an infection, or reactive granulation tissue from an older (2- to 3-week) process. Where appropriate, myelographic contrast may better define the craniocaudal extent of an epidural mass or compromise or compression of the thecal sac, although inflammatory masses encroaching on the cord or nerve roots frequently are adequately defined on studies with intravenous contrast alone.[23]

Diagnostic drainage or biopsy, which is necessary to confirm the diagnosis and identify the responsible agents, can be guided by CT. The adequacy of percutaneous or surgical drainage of associated abscesses can be assessed. With time and treatment, sequential studies should show soft tissue masses decreasing and reactive osteosclerosis appearing. Occasional paravertebral calcifications will appear, particularly with tuberculous infections.[23,24]

Although the incidence of tubercular infections is decreasing, tuberculosis remains the most common agent of vertebral infection. Infectious spondylitis remains the most common of such infections.[26] Frequently a more indolent process than pyogenic infection, spondylitis may be an unsuspected diagnosis, or may be more extensive at the time of CT than plain films or symptoms had indicated. Certain features may suggest a tubercular rather than pyogenic osteomyelitis. As with pyogenic infections, the lower spine is the most common site, but tuberculosis may show a greater disposition to involve the cervical spine as well. The tubercular spondylitis tends to be associated with extensive paraspinous masses or cold abscesses, which may show dense rim enhancement and variable calcifications.[23] Like some fungal infections, tuberculosis may travel

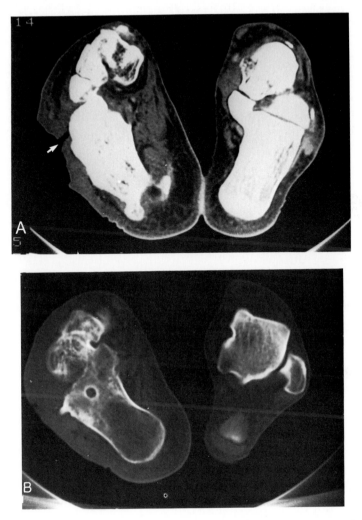

FIG. 4-8.   (A) Chronic osteomyelitis in a 36-year-old man with a history of childhood polio and subsequent subtalar fusion. He had a 6-week history of pain and swelling with more recent development of a large blisterlike collection over the lateral right foot. When unroofed in the emergency room, this ulcer wept pus and bone debris. Plantar plane noncontrast CT at soft tissue windows demonstrated diffuse soft tissue swelling and blurring of tissue planes in comparison to the normal left. A sinus tract (arrow) penetrates to bone from the floor of the ulcer crater. (B) Noncontrast CT, plantar plane, just distal to (A). Bone windows demonstrate a cystic cavity of the distal calcaneous surrounded by sclerotic bone, compatible with surgically proven chronic osteomyelitis with abscess cavity, believed to be the source of the sequestrae and bone debris obtained at drainage.

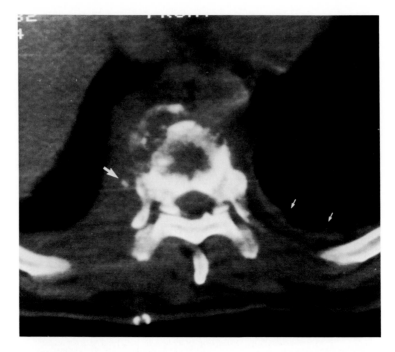

FIG. 4-9. Marked vertebral body destruction is seen with sparing of the posterior elements in a 65-year-old man with osteomyelitis of T-10. Small fragments of bone are seen in the right paravertebral mass (arrow). Some pleural reaction can be seen posteriorly on the left (small arrows).

along the anterior or, less commonly, posterior paraspinous ligaments, allowing involvement of contiguous or, less freqently, more distant vertebral bodies without necessarily involving the intervening disc. Multicentric hematogenous infection may create the same picture. With contiguous body infection, the disc is destroyed approximately 50 percent of the time.[26] In comparison to pyogenic infections, there is a greater propensity towards localizing in the vertebral body rather than the posterior elements, and in the anterior portion of the vertebral body rather than the posterior.[23]

Sacroiliac Joint

The obliquely oriented sacroiliac joint, buried in soft tissue and bone and having a complex curved surface, can be difficult to image in cases of suspected sacroiliitis or infection. Even with special radiographic views, conventional radiographs of the abnormal sacroiliac joint can be disappointing. Subchondral textural changes or alteration in joint width may take 2 to 3 weeks to be seen on plain film. Radionuclide studies are positive earlier, but remain very nonspecific and give little anatomic detail. Thin-section tomography may be more informative, especially in cases of sacroiliitis but requires relatively high radiation doses (3.6 to 6.48 rad per examination).[27]

Computed tomography has several advantages over these imaging modalities.

As with any complex three-dimensional structure, the sacroiliac joint is ideally visualized by CT, with subtle alterations of both topography and density being demonstrated. Focal osteopenia or bony resorption will be seen, as will reactive sclerosis or hyperostosis. Erosions may be seen with active joint inflammation, and need to be distinguished from the normal insertional "pits" of the sacral ligaments seen in the ligamentous compartment (cephalad and dorsal, with bilateral symmetry).[28] CT is particularly sensitive to alterations in joint width, sclerosis, and intra-articular ankylosis.[29] CT may better define a process as primary septic arthritis (involvement of joint cartilage and bone along both sides of the joint, simultaneously) or osteomyelitis with secondary joint involvement (unilateral bone involvement first, followed by joint and finally apposing bone involvement). Osteomyelitis, whether primary or secondary to septic arthritis (Figs. 4-11, 4-12), will be seen earlier than on plain films. Asymmetry

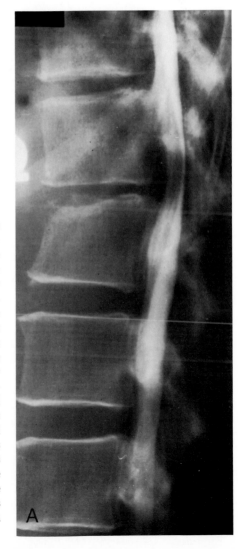

FIG. 4-10. (A) In a 57-year-old diabetic woman with surgically proven osteomyelitis and paravertebral abscess at T-12 to L-1, myelography shows disc space narrowing, depression of the anterior superior endplate of L-1, and destruction of underlying bone. An extradural mass displaces the ventral aspect of the thecal sac. (B) Transaxial CT following metrizamide myelography. There is destruction of the anterior portion of the T-12 vertebral body with fragmented bone in the right paravertebral tissues (arrows). The extradural mass compressing the ventral thecal sac was believed to be an inflammatory canal mass. (C) Sagittal reconstruction confirms the myelographic and transaxial findings and is the best plane to delineate extensive involvement of the inferior portion of the T-12 vertebral body (arrow), which was not suspected from findings on the plain film.

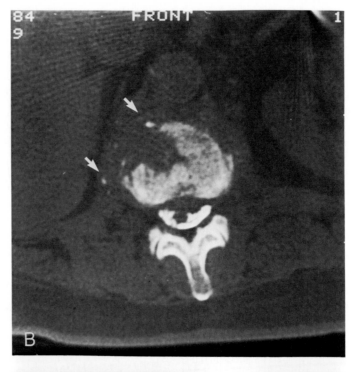

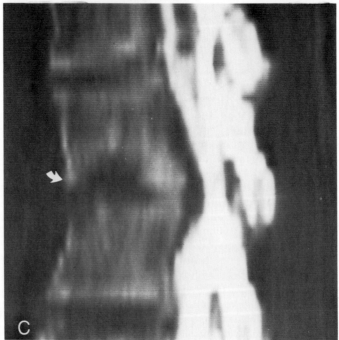

FIG. 4-10. (*Continued*).

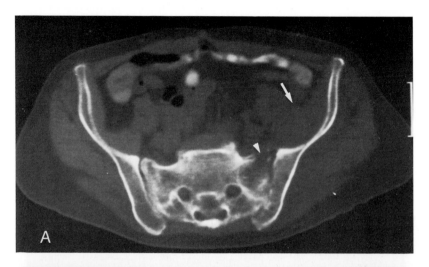

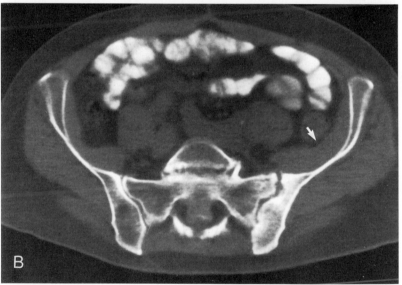

FIG. 4-11. (A) Transaxial CT at the level of S-2 in a 56-year-old man with back pain. Biopsy-proven osteomyelitis with lytic destruction of the left ventral sacral wing, widening of the anterior half of the SI joint, and loss of cortical definition on the iliac articular surface (arrowhead) are noted. There is left iliopsoas swelling (arrow). Although this process crosses the joint, the marked asymmetry of bone involvement supports the diagnosis of primary sacral osteomyelitis with secondary septic arthritis. (B) After 10 weeks of treatment, CT at the level of S-1 shows a widened and irregular left SI joint in comparison to the normal right. There is reactive sclerosis involving both the iliac and sacral subarticular bone. Only minimal residual left iliopsoas prominence remains (arrow).

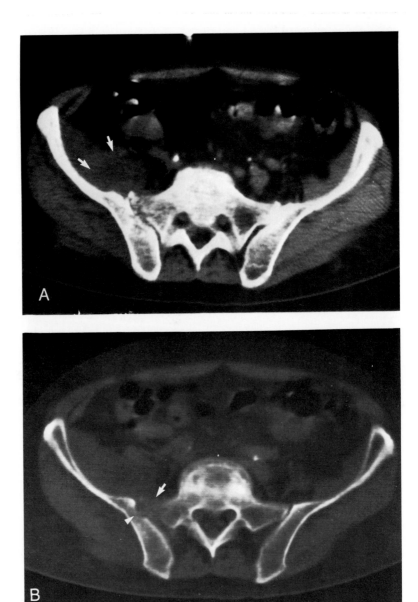

FIG. 4-12. (A) Tuberculosis in a 63-year-old Greek man seeking treatment for back pain. Soft tissue windows show right iliopsoas swelling with a low-attenuation collection medially (arrows) that proved to be a tubercular abscess. There is irregularity and widening of the ventral portion of the right SI joint. (B) Bone windows better define lytic destruction of the right sacral wing (arrow) with more focal erosion and destruction on the iliac side of the joint (arrowhead).

of the muscles in the iliac fossa may be one of the earlier signs of septic arthritis and/or osteomyelitis. There may be loss of definition of soft tissue planes, with soft tissue distortion and edema in early stages and, in some cases, frank fluid collection or abscess later. Associated soft tissue abnormalities such as abscess (with or without gas accumulation) are defined and, where indicated, CT will provide interventional guidance for percutaneous drainage or diagnostic biopsy of such collections.

Both the sensitivity and specificity of sacroiliac CT are superior to those of plain films. CT in this setting, as elsewhere, tends to be more definitive and to document more extensive abnormalities than can be appreciated by other modalities. Depending on technique and collimation, the radiation dose is usually 1.5 to 3 rads, which is far less than tomography and represents a lower gonadal dose than conventional plain film tomography.[28] (Beck TJ, personal communication.) Additional high-resolution images can be obtained on an individual basis at critical levels, but routine scanning parameters usually suffice.

The oblique lie of the sacroiliac joint allows good definition on transaxial images, with characteristic changes in the appearance of the normal joint with cephalocaudal and dorsoventral progression.[28] We do not angle the gantry for routine SI studies. However, multiplanar reconstructions, particularly in the coronal plane, contribute to a more thorough visualization of the sacroiliac joint. On both transaxial and reconstructed views, the contralateral, frequently normal, side usually is available for comparison, thus increasing our appreciation of subtle alterations in contour or density. Acute inflammation will create local osteopenia and focal erosions, with more chronic inflammation being accompanied by reactive sclerosis. The joint space may show areas of either widening or narrowing that can be best appreciated when compared to the contralateral side.

REFERENCES

1. Waldvogel FA, Medoff G, Swartz MM: Osteomyelitis: a review of clinical features. Therapeutic considerations and unusual aspects. N Engl J Med 282(4):198, 1970
2. Resnick D, Niwayama G (eds): Diagnosis of Bone and Joint Disorders, Vol. 1, p. 652. WB Saunders, Philadelphia, 1981
3. Wyngaarden FJB, Smith LH (eds): Cecil Textbook of Medicine, 16th edition. WB Saunders, Philadelphia, 1982
4. Hadjis NS, Carr DH, Banks L, Pflug JJ: The role of CT in the diagnosis of primary lymphedema of the lower limb. AJR 144:361, 1985
5. Gamba JL, Silverman PM, Ling D et al: Primary lower extremity lymphedema: CT diagnosis. Radiology 149:218, 1983
6. Weinstein L, Barza MA: Gas gangrene. N Engl J Med 289:1129, 1977
7. Vukanicoviac S, Hauser H, Wettstein O: Myonecrosis induced by drug overdose: pathogenesis, clinical aspects and radiological manifestations. Eur J Radiol 3:314, 1983
8. Feingold DS: Gangrenous and crepitant cellulitis. J Am Acad Dermatol 6:289, 1982
9. Ramirez H, Jr., Brown JD, Evans JW: Case report 225. Skel Radiol 9:223, 1983

10. Vukanovic S, Hauser H, Wettstein P: CT localization of myonecrosis for surgical decompression. AJR 135:1298, 1980

11. Kahn DS, Pritzker KPH: The pathophysiology of bone infection. Clin Orthop Rel Res 96:12, 1973

12. Mundy GR, Raisz LG, Shapiro JL et al: Big and little forms of osteoclast activating factor. J Clin Invest 60:122, 1977

13. Rosen RA, Morehouse HT, Karp HJ, Yu GSM: Intracortical fissuring in Osteomyelitis. Radiology 141:17, 1981

14. Edeiken J: Roentgen Diagnosis of Diseases of Bone, 3rd edition. Williams and Wilkins, Baltimore, 1981

15. Kuhn JP, Berger PE: Computed tomographic diagnosis of osteomyelitis. Radiology 130:503, 1979

16. Hermann G, Rose JS, Strauss L: Tumor infiltration of bone marrow: Comparative study using computed tomography. Skel Radiol 11:17, 1984

17. Ram PC, Martinez S, Karobkin M et al: CT detection of intraosseous gas: a new sign of ostomyelitis. AJR 137:721, 1981

18. Rafii M, Firooznia H, Golimbu C, McCauley DI: Hematogenous osteomyelitis with fat-fluid level shown by CT. Radiology 153:493, 1984

19. Wing VW, Jeffrey RB, Jr., Federle MP et al: Chronic osteomyelitis examined by CT. Radiology 154:171, 1985

20. Seltzer SE: Value of computed tomography in planning medical and surgical treatment of chronic osteomyelitis. J Comput Assist Tomogr 8(3):482, 1984

21. Sapico FL, Montgomerie JZ: Vertebral osteomyelitis in intravenous drug abusers. Report of three cases and review of the literature. Rev Infect Dis 2:196, 1980

22. Hermann G, Mendelson DS, Cohen BA, Train JS: Role of computed tomography in the diagnosis of infections spondylitis. J Comput Assist Tomogr 7(6):961, 1983

23. Whelan MA, Naidich DP, Post JD, Chase NE: Computed tomography of spinal tuberculosis. J Comput Assist Tomogr 7(1):25, 1983

24. Golimbu C, Firooznia H, Rafii M: CT of osteomyelitis of the spine. AJR 142:159, 1984

25. Glenn WV, Jr., Rhodes ML, Altschuler ER et al: Multiplanar display computerized body tomography applications in the lumbar spine. Spine 4:282, 1979

26. LaBerge JM, Brant-Zawadzki M: Evaluation of Pott's disease with computed tomography. Neuroradiology 26:429, 1984

27. De Smet AA, Gardner JD, Lindsley HB et al: Tomography for evaluation of sacroiliitis. AJR 139:577, 1982

28. Kozin F, Carrera GF, Ryan LM et al: Computed tomography of the sacroiliac joints: comparison with complex-motion tomography. J Comput Assist Tomogr 8(1):31, 1984

5 Assessment of Musculoskeletal Trauma

DONNA MAGID
ELLIOT K. FISHMAN

Computed tomography has become the study of choice in the evaluation of the traumatized patient. It permits rapid and relatively noninvasive imaging of the full spectrum of traumatic injuries, whether to the central nervous system, thorax, viscera, or musculoskeletal system. The severely traumatized patient can be studied with only minimal positioning maneuvers. With careful positioning, comparison to the contralateral side can be used to augment appreciation of subtle abnormalities. Manipulation of acquired data allows better definition of soft tissue and of bone. Soft tissue injuries may be mapped with a precision unavailable with any other imaging modality. Fractures missed or poorly appreciated on plain film may be detected. Complex and multiple fractures can be thoroughly defined, allowing better triage into treatment modalities. The postoperative patient who experiences unexpected pain or loss of range of motion in the recovery period can be assessed for true status of reduction and healing. Long-term follow-up can confirm healing or identify posttraumatic complications such as degenerative arthritis, nonunion, and avascular necrosis.

This chapter reviews our experience in evaluating musculoskeletal trauma, and will describe specific areas where CT is most helpful. The importance of meticulous imaging protocols, including multiplanar reconstructions (multiplanar reconstruction and display, MPR/D), are discussed.

TECHNIQUE

Certain constant general principles of technique can be modified as necessary to fit the specific anatomy of interest and the individual situation. Ideally, patient instruction and positioning encourage compliance by ensuring patient comfort, and guarantee sufficient symmetry to allow comparison to the contralateral side. In general, patients are positioned supine and in the anatomic position, with arms symmetrically elevated from the area of interest if necessary. For studies of the foot or lower leg, the feet may be positioned closest to the gantry; otherwise, patients are positioned head-first. Feet are in neutral position and together. Small pillows for support are provided behind the knee or as necessary. Particularly in those patients in whom MPR is advisable, the feet, knees, and, as indicated, shoulders and elbows, may be taped to discourage any random motion between scans. When possible, instruction is given to reinforce the importance of remaining motionless, and to allow uniform end-expiratory phase scanning. Intravenous contrast is not required routinely for the musculoskeletal exam, although it is frequently used as part of an overall screening exam of the traumatized liver, spleen, kidney, and other organs.

Routine scanning parameters (230 mAs, 3.2 sec, 125 kVp) are used. Slice collimation and interval are determined by the area of interest; while 8-mm slices at 8-mm intervals may be adequate to assess large areas such as the sacroiliac (SI) joint or iliac wing, contiguous 4-mm slices are advisable through smaller structures such as the glenoid or the sternoclavicular joint. Any observed abnormality should be "bracketed," scanned superiorly and inferiorly to extend past the apparent abnormality and into more normal tissue. Frequently the initial musculoskeletal exam is performed as part of a comprehensive emergency evaluation, and as such, areas such as the SI joint or acetabular dome initially may be surveyed with 8-mm collimation at 8-mm intervals. For questionable abnormalities of deep structures (e.g., sacrum or SI joint), additional selected high-resolution (5.2 sec, 450 mAs, 2- or 4-mm collimation) images may be obtained. When abnormalities are detected by an initial screening examination and/or once the patient has been stabilized, these areas of interest may be restudied using multiplanar technique. Multiplanar reconstruction protocols require thin overlapping slices (4-mm collimation at 3-mm intervals) with stringent attention to positioning and to instructions and taping to counter motion. Even minor toe-wiggling between slices can generate aliasing (line or zigzag) artifacts on the reconstructions. A full discussion of the MPR/D examination including technique can be found in Chapter 10.

SPECIFIC APPLICATIONS

Sternoclavicular Joint

The sternoclavicular (SC) joint is a diarthrodial saddle joint with a small bony articular surface. Less than half of the medial clavicular surface articulates with the clavicular notch of the sternum. This joint is therefore dependent on the enveloping ligaments for its structural integrity. These are of sufficient strength and stability so as to make SC joint dislocation a relatively uncommon injury. Motor vehicle accidents are the primary cause, with sports injuries responsible for most of the remaining fractures and dislocations. The relatively benign anterior dislocation is more common than either the posterior or retrosternal dislocation, either of which can jeopardize the immediately underlying mediastinal structures.[1,2] While fractures of the medial clavicle may be less subtle on plain film than dislocation, the two injuries may be associated and the complete diagnosis can be difficult to document. Such fracture–dislocations are most commonly associated with steering wheel trauma, implying sufficient transmission of force to put the underlying mediastinum and great vessels at risk.

Conventional roentgenographic evaluation of the SC joint can be frustrating. The cortices involved are relatively thin, and the joints are oriented obliquely.[3] While conventional wisdom dictates the general principal of obtaining two views of 90° to rule out fracture, this is virtually impossible for this joint. Comparison to the allegedly normal contralateral side is impossible on the special views. Superimposition of the underlying thoracic structures further limits imaging options. Therefore, CT is the ideal imaging modality, being both simple and accurate.[2,3]

The SC joint is a small structure and should be studied with contiguous 4-mm slices. Specific breathing instructions must be given for consistent positioning, with breath-holding at end-expiration being very reproducible ("Breath in, breath out, relax, hold your breath, and don't move . . ."). Intravenous contrast enhancement is essential for those patients in whom history, clinical findings, or plain film findings raise the question of mediastinal or vascular trauma. The study can be extended at 8-mm intervals caudad or cephalad as necessary to follow suspected mediastinal abnormalities.

Computed tomography allows clear visualization of the SCJ with the contralateral side for comparison. Bony integrity can be defined, as can subtle fractures and dislocation (Fig. 5-1). Where indicated by history, symptoms, or anatomic findings, underlying mediastinum and great vessel anatomy may be sufficiently defined to replace or defer the aortogram in the severely traumatized but apparently stable patient. The overlying soft tissues and muscle planes are defined, again using the contralateral side for comparison. Interposed bone fragments or soft tissue that might preclude reduction can also be demonstrated.

Scapula and Shoulder

The scapula is a flat bone, the enveloping muscles of which provide both protective cushioning and rich vascular supply. Fractures of the scapular body and spine therefore most commonly result from significant direct trauma and often are associated with other injuries to the bony thorax, shoulder girdle, or spine. If these other injuries are severe, the scapular fracture initially may be overlooked. Fractures of the scapular neck are rare, usually separating the glenoid and coracoid as distal fragment(s).[1] Associated with up to 20 percent of traumatic shoulder dislocations, glenoid fractures are among the most common scapular fractures. The glenoid is a shallow cavity requiring (among other features) an intact and attached cartilaginous labrum for joint stability. Even an apparently small bony fragment, therefore, can imply a larger—and significant—cartilaginous tear, impairing function and increasing the risk of dislocation.

The normal shoulder is the most mobile joint in the body, and as a result, a number of special views have been developed to improve plain film assess-

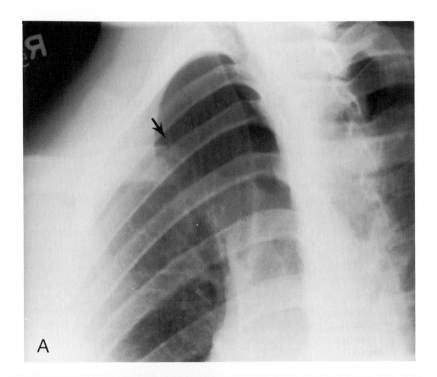

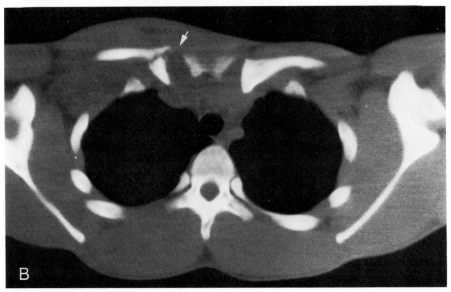

FIG. 5-1. (A) Sternoclavicular view of an 18-year-old man with fracture of the right medial clavicle shows discontinuity of the superior cortex (arrow) but poorly defines the SC joint. (B) Noncontrast CT scan of this lesion confirms the fracture and reveals subtle widening of the right sternoclavicular joint (arrow) in comparison to the normal left. There is only minimal posterior displacement of the medial fragment and the underlying mediastinal structures appear normal. Chest wall soft tissue swelling is noted.

ment. However, even if pain and injury do not preclude adequate positioning, conventional imaging is limited by the fact that the shoulder and scapula are complex three-dimensional structures superimposed against the larger and equally complex thorax.

Computed tomography provides a better overview of the scapula, shoulder (discussed in more detail in Chapter 7), and related structures. Careful positioning and breathing instructions ensure bilateral symmetry for comparison and minimize respiratory motion. The arms are placed at the patient's side, with the hands supinated. If multiplanar reconstructions are to be performed, the arms are taped above the elbow to discourage motion.

Transaxial CT again removes the element of superimposition and allows detailed delineation of bone, joint, and associated soft tissue, with the contralateral side for comparison. Air or positive-contrast arthrography may improve definition of the cartilaginous labrum on CT[4] (see Chap. 7). Subtle injuries missed on plain films, such as shear fractures of the humeral head, nondisplaced scapular fractures, or small avulsions off the glenoid or coracoid, may be detected. Fracture fragment position and rotation will be noted as will any interposed soft tissue fragment or foreign matter that might compromise reduction (Figs. 5-2 to 5-4). The addition of MPR refines the mapping of abnormal anatomy, demonstrating the structures and relationships of interest in three dimensions (Fig. 5-4). Small glenoid or coracoid avulsions may be better seen on reconstructions as are some displaced fracture fragments. Yet MPR/D tends to be of more limited use in the shoulder, since even with careful positioning and immobilization, respiratory and cardiac motion between scans may degrade the reformatted images of some patients.

Pelvis and Sacrum

A number of pelvic trauma classification systems have been developed, with the most useful being based on stability and implying prognosis rather than emphasizing the mechanism of injury. Whatever the classification system, minor fractures are stable and carry a good prognosis, and include such injuries as isolated fractures of the ilium, unilateral pubic ramus fracture, and avulsion fractures. The major fractures are unstable, with a significant morbidity and mortality, and usually include fractures of the acetabulum, double vertical hemipelvis (Malgaigne), sacrum, or bilateral ramae.[1] More than 80 percent of pelvic fractures are the results of motor vehicle accidents, with the rest accounted for by falls and crush injuries.

The sacrum is a thick and convoluted structure with relatively thin cortex, pierced by the central sacral canal and four paired dorsal and ventral sacral foramina.[5] Even with special positioning, information provided by conventional radiographs may be limited by foreshortening due to curvature on frontal view, the enormous bulk of superimposed soft tissue on the lateral view, by the inability to obtain views at 90° to each other, and by overlying bowel gas and feces. The patient with severe osteoporosis may also receive a suboptimal plain film examination, and the severely traumatized patient may be unwilling

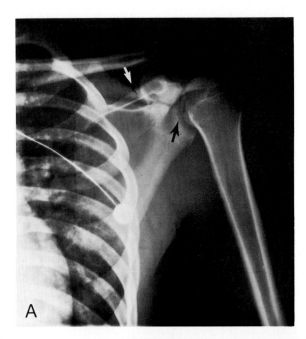

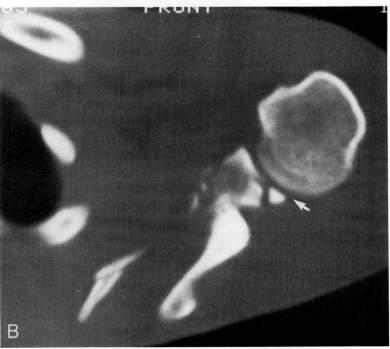

FIG. 5-2. (A) Radiograph of 23-year-old man with comminuted fracture of the scapular neck involving the coracoid and extending into the glenoid (arrows). (b) Transaxial CT confirms involvement of glenohumeral joint (arrow), and at this and other levels defined a relatively nondisplaced comminuted fracture of the neck and body, with the coracoid separated as an anterior fragment.

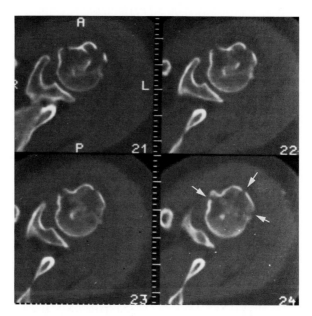

FIG. 5-3. A fracture of the humeral head of a 63-year-old woman struck by motor vehicle was seen on initial plain films. Transaxial CT scan defined a nondisplaced four-part fracture of the proximal humurus (arrows), sparing the glenohumeral joint.

or unable to comply with positioning maneuvers. The SI joint, like the sacrum, is curved, oblique, and deep, making CT the optimal imaging modality.[6] Comparison to the contralateral SI joint can increase the sensitivity of CT, since slight asymmetry is increasingly common with age but normally is not seen in patients under 30 years[7] (Figs. 5-5 to 5-7).

In the stable patient with unclear symptoms and indeterminate findings on plain films, CT can reveal previously occult injuries. While a number of special plain film views have been developed to assess the bony pelvis, CT offers the simplest and most thorough means of investigating both bony and visceral pelvic trauma. The severely traumatized patient requires rapid and sensitive assessment to characterize bony trauma and associated injuries, which CT can provide without extensive, painful, and potentially risky repositioning maneuvers. This simplicity of positioning protects the patient in traction or with suspected visceral damage or internal hemorrhage. The addition of multiplanar reconstructions gives superb and therapeutically relevant mapping of the sacrum, sacroiliac joint, acetabulum, and hip.

Even when comminuted, the isolated iliac wing fracture can be a surprisingly benign lesion. Most commonly these are the result of a lateral compression injury, folding the wing forward. Although the area has rich blood supply, the tendency of muscle pull to contain and replace the fragments laterally may protect the major arteries and viscera. An isolated fracture is considered a stable injury. CT will demonstrate the degree of wing displacement or rotation, position of smaller fragments, and associated soft tissue and muscular trauma (Fig. 5-8).

Frequently these fractures are part of a more complex injury extending into

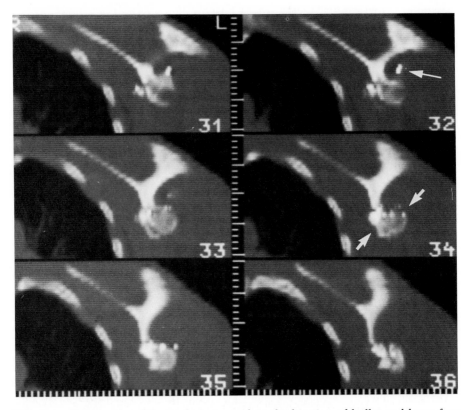

FIG. 5-4. Preoperative CT was done to confirm the location of bullet and bone fragments in a 28-year-old man with a gun shot wound to the left shoulder. Fragments were seen on coronal reconstructions (sequence is anterior to posterior) to be well-localized in the axillary portion of the body of the scapula (paired arrows) and inferior to the acromial spine (arrow).

the acetabulum or SI joint, or compromising the pelvic ring. Accurate anatomic assessment and restoration are required to minimize the morbidity of pelvic ring disruptions.[8,9] CT removes the element of superimposition limiting demonstration of plain film anatomy; it clarifies the degree of comminution and precise fragment position, and demonstrates subtle fracture lines and diastases (Fig. 5-9, 5-10A). The unstable hemipelvis may displace along three planes, and frequently includes a rotatory component. CT also defines the posterior pelvic ring, an area inadequately visualized on plain films.[10] Closed or open reduction and, where applicable, internal fixation can be both planned and assessed posttherapeutically with CT.

We have had several cases where CT and CT/MPR provided unexpected findings, particularly subtle SI diastasis, extension of fracture into the acetabulum or SI joint, and sacral fracture. Subtle anterior or posterior iliac displacement across a diastatic SI joint may be otherwise undetectable, but carries prognostic

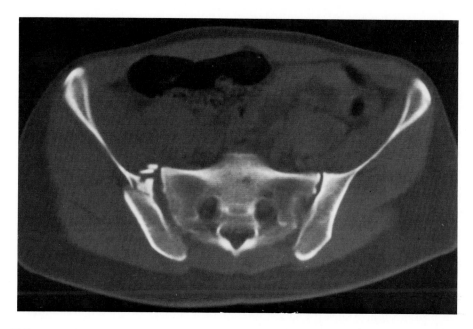

FIG. 5-5. CT scan of a 16-year-old girl with nondisplaced iliac fracture extending into a widely diastatic right SI joint. There is soft tissue swelling. The sacrum is intact.

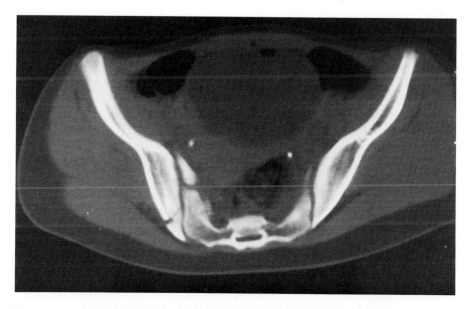

FIG. 5-6. In another 16-year-old girl with right pelvic fracture involving the sacrum and iliac, very subtle diastasis is appreciable only by comparing the two sides at several levels. In an older patient, such a subtle asymmetry could be a normal age-related finding. Soft tissue distortion is minimal.

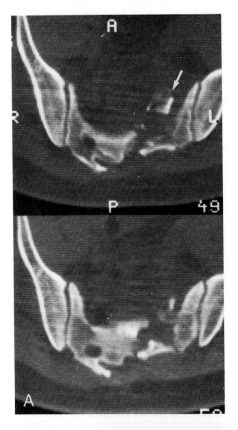

FIG. 5-7. (A) This initial prereduction transaxial study of a 36-year-old man with a comminuted fracture of the left sacrum involving the neural foramina shows subtle anterior displacement of the left pelvis, and anterior displacement of one large fracture fragment (arrow). (B) The same patient after 10 days of traction (hardware creates artifact). Only minimal reduction has been obtained. The fragments are still distracted (arrows). There continues to be mild left SI diastasis in comparison to the normal right side, and minimal anterior displacement of the hemipelvis. The patient underwent surgery for open reduction internal fixation.

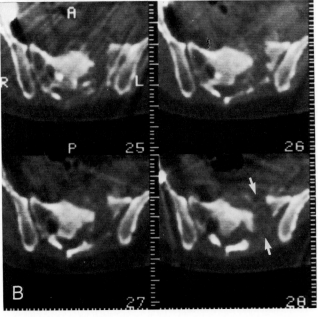

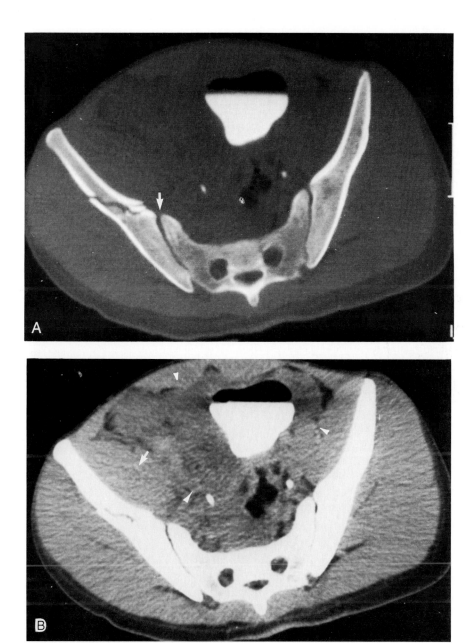

FIG. 5-8.   (A) Iliac wing fracture in a 28-year-old man who fell from a building. Bone windows show a comminuted but nondisplaced right iliac wing fracture. There is subtle SI joint asymmetry, with minimal widening of the ventral aspect on the right (arrow). (B) Soft tissue windows demonstrate that the right iliopsoas muscle is enlarged (arrow). Hematoma (arrowheads) surrounds and displaces the bladder and minimally displaces the right ureter.

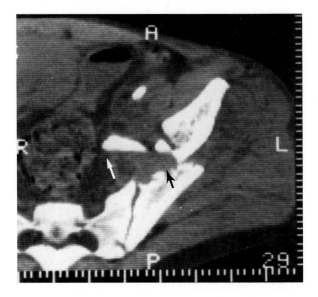

FIG. 5-9. Findings in a 51-year-old man with left iliac and acetabular fractures and mild SI diastasis. The iliac wing fracture is comminuted, with external rotation of the major lateral fragment and medial displacement of two major fragments potentially threatening bowel (white arrow) and other soft tissues. Interposed tissue and/or hematoma (black arrow) may compromise closed reduction.

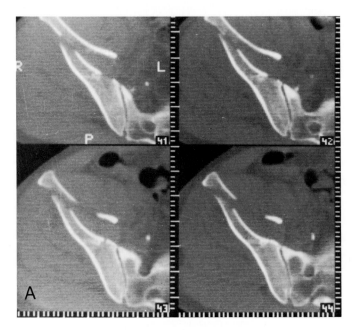

FIG. 5-10. (A) The iliac wing is externally rotated in this 45-year-old man with iliac fracture extending into the acetabulum. The SI joint was intact.

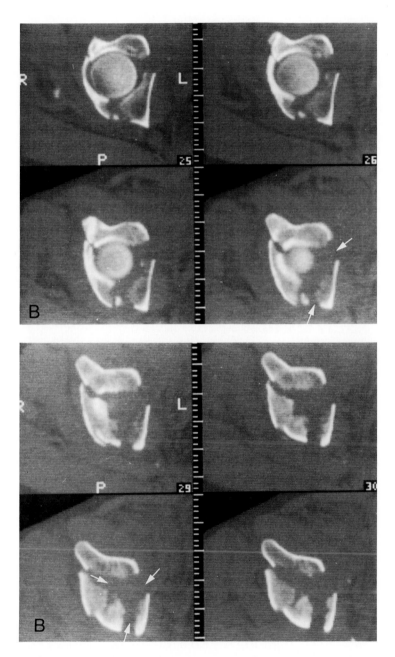

FIG. 5-10. (*continued*)   (B) Eight transaxial images progressing superiorly from the mid-femoral head to the acetabular dome demonstrate a complex right acetabular "T" fracture, with displaced fractures through the anterior, posterior, and medial components creating a gap in the acetabular dome (arrows).

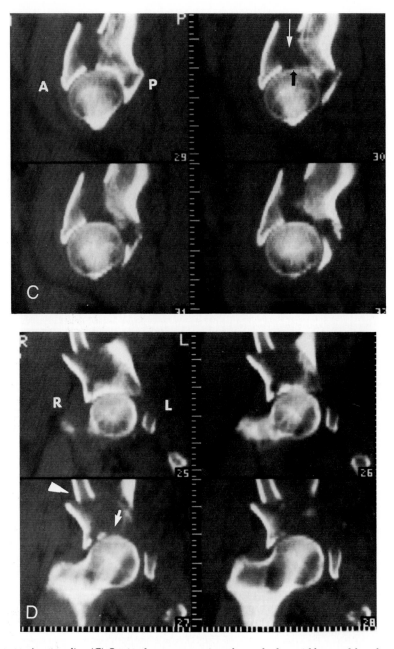

FIG. 5-10. (*continued*)   (C) Sagittal reconstruction through the midfemoral head confirms the wide gap in the superior aspect of the weight-bearing surface (black arrow) caused by the separation of acetabular dome fragments (white arrow). Both the joint surface discontinuity and the loss of dome support are indications for open reduction internal fixation. The posterior column fracture shows minimal displacement of the inferior fragment. (D) Coronal images through the midfemoral head confirm the loss of joint surface (arrow) and dome support, showing iliac wing displacement (arrowhead) corresponding to that seen on transaxial image (A).

significance (Fig. 5-7, 5-11A). The definition of comminution and of fragment position guide and frequently alter therapeutic decisions and surgical planning. Multiplanar reconstructions at the level of the SI joint provide superior assessment of joint integrity and of iliac and sacral fractures involving the joint (Fig. 5-11). The potential area of interest for reformatting (128 pixels) suffices to include the contralateral SI joint, allowing comparison for symmetry of width and contour. The patient's age must be considered in assessing slight SI asymmetry, which increases with age.[7] Coronal reconstructions are particularly useful, imaging along the cephalocaudal extent of both SI joints and transecting the foramina at 2-mm increments to look for subtle diastasis or fractures. The primary contribution of the sagittal views in this context is in determining the degree and direction of fragment displacement and rotation.[11] Caution must be taken to recognize the normal regional variation in SI joint structure as scanning progresses cephalocaudal and anteroposteriorly; the inclusion of the contralateral side aids in distinguishing normal geographic variation in morphology from subtle pathologic change.[11,12]

Acetabulum

The acetabulum can be described as an arch formed by the supporting anterior and posterior columns and bridged by the dome segments. The combination of complicated anatomy, frequently comminuted fractures, and inadequate plain film definition traditionally has made the acetabular fracture a difficult management problem. There are a number of classification systems, with the most useful being those that carry therapeutic and prognostic significance. The "personality"[9] of the fracture is determined predominantly by division into simple (isolated, of a single column or the medial wall) or complex fractures. The latter is more common and requires further definition of degree of comminution, fragment displacement, and rotation.[9] For healing with an acceptable pain-free range of motion and capacity for weight-bearing, there must be an adequately congruent joint surface and sufficient weight-bearing support. The key weight-bearing structures are the acetabular dome, the relatively small anterior column, and the more robust posterior column. Femoral head dislocation, most common with posterior column fracture, requires prompt reduction to decrease the risk of avascular necrosis. Extension of the fracture into the iliac wing and/or SI joint affects prognosis, since associated fragment rotation and increased instability will make reduction even more difficult to achieve and maintain.

Routine transaxial imaging is used to examine the iliac wings, anterior and posterior columns, the medial wall and cotyloid fossa, the joint space and the femoral head, as well as all the surrounding soft tissue. This may define the presence and extent of fracture or dislocation, degree of comminution and of joint disruption (in terms of both disrupted support integrity and joint surface discongruity), and suggest the presence of intra-articular fragments or fragments impinging on the bladder or other viscera (Fig. 5-10B). Even with thin slices, however, partial volume effect compromises assessment of the superior pole of the femur and the superior portion of the joint. Transaxial imaging alone does not convey adequately the degree to which the dome and columns have been disrupted by trauma.

Therefore we routinely perform CT with MPR/D on any patient with clinical or radiographic evidence of acetabular trauma, or with acetabular fracture detected on an initial posttraumatic screening CT. The addition of sagittal and coronal reformations provides superior visualization of the key weight-bearing structures: the superior pole of the femur, the columns, the acetabular dome, and the joint surfaces (Fig. 5-10C,D). Discontinuity (fragment distraction) and discongruity (surface step-offs) of the acetabular side of the joint line are best displayed on reformatted images (Fig. 5-12). While transaxial scans will document fractures of the anterior and posterior columns and acetabular dome, it remains for sagittal and coronal images to define the extent to which the integrity of these structures has been compromised. The surgeon can best consider the degree to which congruity and weight-bearing support have been lost, confirm the presence of intraarticular fragments suggested on transaxial views, and plan for anatomic restoration when reformatted images supplement routine

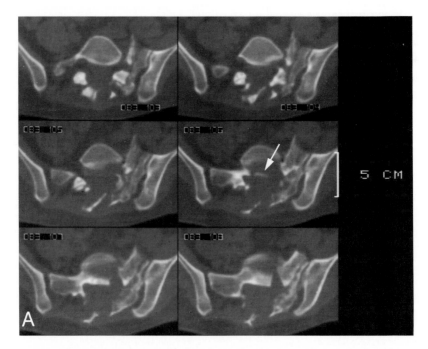

FIG. 5-11. (A) Transaxial CT of a 36-year-old woman with sacral fractures poorly seen on initial radiographic examination shows a comminuted sacral fracture, here seen at the S-1 level, allowing anterior shift of the entire hemipelvis. There is some left posterior SI diastasis. The fracture disrupts the central neural canal, with one fragment protruding into the canal (arrow).

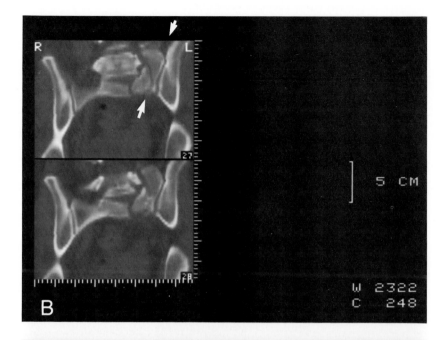

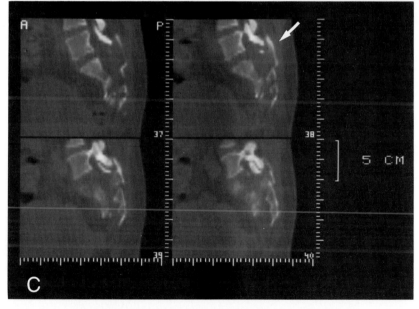

FIG. 5-11. (*continued*)   (B) Coronal reconstructions through the sacrum confirm the position of fractures and fragments and demonstrate cephalad displacement of the left hemipelvis (arrows). This far anteriorly, only minimal widening of the inferior left S-I joint can be appreciated. (C) Sagittal reconstructions show posterior displacement of sacral fragments (arrow).

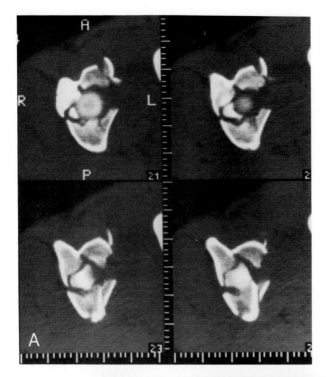

FIG. 5-12. (A,B) Thin (4-mm) slices through the superior pole of the femur and superior aspect of the joint space of a young man show complex acetabular dome fracture, which is better characterized on the sagittal reconstruction (B). The extent of joint surface and acetabular dome discontinuity (arrows) are better defined, as is a nondisplaced posterior column fracture (arrowhead).

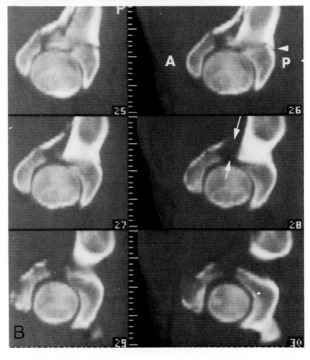

transaxial views (Fig. 5-13). If sufficient support and congruity can be documented, conservative management with traction and bed rest may be appropriate. For the candidate for surgery, precise definition of abnormal anatomy influences operative technique, choice of hardware, and postoperative rehabilitation (passive range-of-motion exercises, physical therapy, and progressive weight-bearing).[13]

Our first 40 patients demonstrated the clinical utility of CT/MPR in acetabular fractures.[13] Twelve patients had associated injuries of the femur, ischium, sacrum, sacroiliac joint, or symphysis pubis. Five had bilateral fractures, for a total of 45 acetabular fractures.

In four patients, single-column fractures were defined which had been missed (three) or questionable (one) (Fig. 5-14) on plain film, and in one patient, an occult intertrochanteric fracture was discovered. Five patients arriving at CT with tentatively planned closed management via traction subsequently underwent open reduction and internal fixation as a direct result of CT/MPR. Most likely to alter management plans were revelations of significant displacement of acetabular dome or column fragments, of previously unsuspected intraarticular fragments, of greater discongruity, or of more marked instability than had been anticipated from plain films. Three patients scheduled for surgery prior to CT were able instead to receive more conservative closed management, with CT/MPR documenting better congruity and/or support, or less complex injury, than had been anticipated. A fourth patient's surgery was deferred because of CT/MPR documentation of injury too severely comminuted for adequate internal fixation.

There were 11 postoperative CT/MPR examinations, either to define the true status of reduction and fixation or to evaluate unusual pain or disability in the recovery period. Seven patients proved to have reduction as satisfactory as predicted clinically, while four were shown to have less satisfactory alignment than anticipated (Fig. 5-13C). Previously undocumented postoperative complications included one acetabular nonunion, intraarticular projection of one fracture fragment, avascular necrosis of the femoral head, and inadequate reduction of a posterior fracture dislocation.

While not routinely indicated, postoperative transaxial CT can document the true status of acetabular reduction and confirm femoral head relocation. The addition of MPR contributes more detailed assessment of joint surface congruity and continuity, and of dome and column restoration. This permits development of individualized progressive mobilization and weight-bearing programs, and allows for a more realistic prognosis.

It is also of interest to note that while previously the severe artifacts generated by orthopedic hardware markedly limited postoperative CT, recent developments curtail such image degradation. Metal correction algorithms, edge-enhancing kernals, and reversal to negative mode (black on white) all act to counter transaxial image degradation (the latter, subjectively). The MPR/D program preferentially weights true axial data over random axial artifact data, producing surprisingly good coronal and sagittal images in which image "clean up" far exceeds image degradation due to data loss[14] (Fig. 11C, 15D). Further

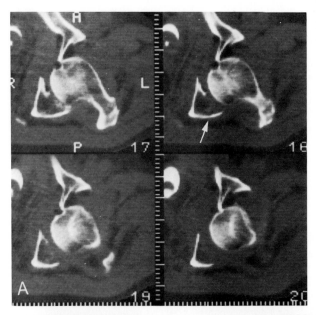

FIG. 5-13. (A) Prereduction transaxial images of a left acetabular fracture with posterior and medial dislocation of the left hip. The posterior column fragment is also displaced and slightly rotated (arrow). (B) Repeat CT was performed following closed reduction and traction. Sagittal reformatted images at the level of the fovea contralis (arrow) show better posterior column position but with a significant gap between fragments disrupting the joint surface and column support (small arrows). This was thought to be an indication for open reduction internal fixation.

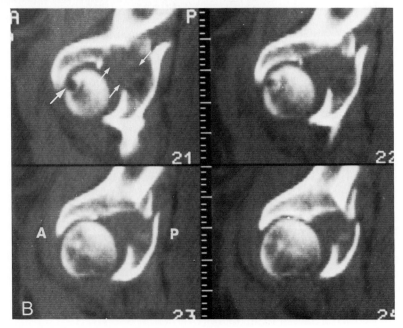

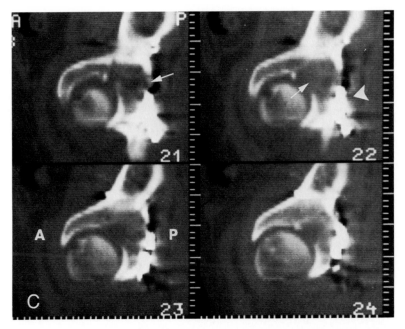

FIG. 5-13. (*continued*) (C) Postoperative CT was performed to confirm reduction. Sagittal reconstructions at the same level show reduction in the joint surface discontinuity and in the posterior column gap (arrows), fixed by screws and plate (arrowhead). Localized hardware artifact only minimally intrudes on assessment of adjacent bone. By documenting the moderate residual joint surface and column deformity, this study allowed the surgeon to design a more conservative progressive mobilization program than had been anticipated initially.

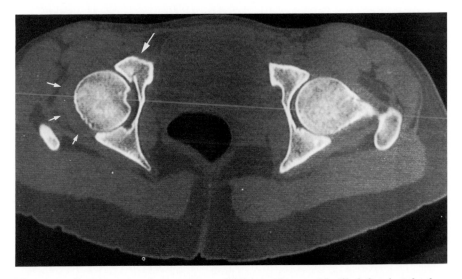

FIG. 5-14. Patient injured in motor vehicle accident, with ill-defined right lower quadrant pain and with a possible acetabular fracture noted on an otherwise normal intravenous urogram. High-resolution transaxial image demonstrated a nondisplaced anterior column fracture (arrow) and a small joint effusion (small arrows).

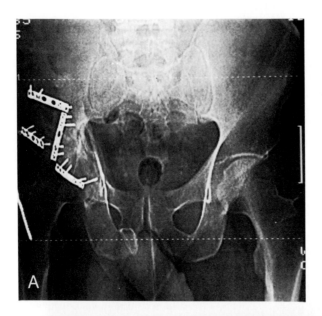

FIG. 5-15. (A) Topogram of a 42-year-old man 10 months after open reduction internal fixation of a right acetabular fracture using four acetabular plates and 16 screws. Patient complained of increasing pain. (B) Transaxial images show some residual deformity of the anterior column (arrowhead) unchanged from previous CT exams. Hardware artifact minimally degrades the posterior column image (arrow).

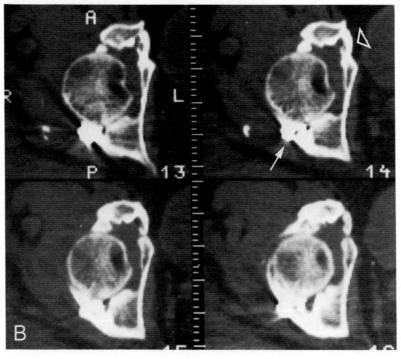

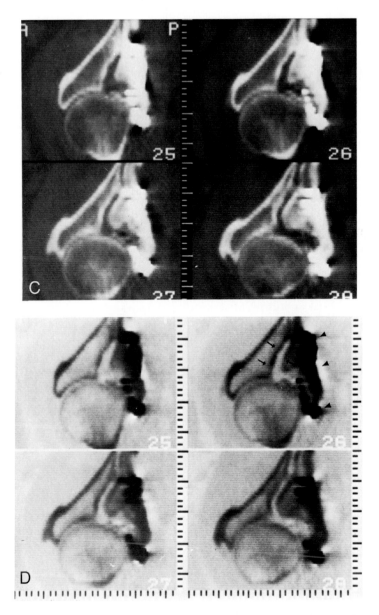

FIG. 5-15. (*continued*)   (C) Sagittal reconstruction shows a vertical fracture line through the acetabular dome, seen on earlier CT exams but now showing a sclerotic margin compatible with nonunion. Although hardware artifact continues to degrade the posterior column image, artifact is well-localized and does not compromise visualization of this change in density of the fracture margin. (D) Reverse-mode sagittal reconstruction can be used to minimize metallic artifact further (arrowheads) and define sclerotic nonunion through the acetabular dome (arrows). This apparent artifact reduction is subjective and viewer-dependent.

image improvement can be expected as the use of titanium implants, rather than higher-attenuation chrome cobalt or stainless steel, increases.[15]

STRESS FRACTURES

The apparently negative history and subtle radiographic appearance of stress fracture can present a diagnostic dilemma. These fractures represent an imbalance between bone stimulation and reparative response. Stress fractures are divided into two groups: the fatigue fracture, produced by abnormal activity in the patient with normal bone; and the insufficiency fracture, which can be seen when normal forces are applied to the patient with bone pathology (e.g., osteoporosis, Paget's disease, or renal osteodystrophy). The fatigue fracture classically is produced by the enthusiastic adoption of a new and repetitive physical activity (e.g., jogging, marching, or break dancing). Muscle tone may increase more rapidly than bone strength in response to such an activity, increasing the unaccustomed forces acting on bone. In response to Wolff's law, these forces induce remodeling, which commences with osteoclastic resorption of lamellar bone. Osteoblastic reactive repair and reinforcement lag behind. This discrepancy creates a vulnerable period, during which time strenuous activity can produce cortical microfractures. Progression to complete fracture can be seen if activity continues to outstrip repair.[16-18]

Radionuclide bone scan, as a rule, is positive by the time of presentation, but may not distinguish between stress fracture, early osteomyelitis, or neoplasm. Findings on conventional radiographs may be unremarkable in the symptomatic patient, since resorption and repair may take as long as 10 to 21 days to produce sufficient alteration in density to be detectable.[16,17,19]

Technique

Careful positioning allows comparison to the asymptomatic side. No intravenous contrast is needed. If no specific area of interest has been localized by plain film, the clinical region of interest is scanned with 4-mm collimation at contiguous intervals. Once a more specific area of interest has been defined, high-resolution technique and 2- to 4-mm slices will best define subtle alterations in texture and density. All images are reviewed at both bone and soft tissue settings; wider than usual bone windows may be used to concentrate on subtle cortical alterations.

Results

Particularly in the presence of a normal contralateral comparison, CT can detect and characterize subtle alterations in the radiodensity of bone, marrow, and surrounding soft tissue (Figs. 5-16, 5-17). Adjacent soft tissue edema may be seen. Subtle callous formation may be defined along both the endosteal and

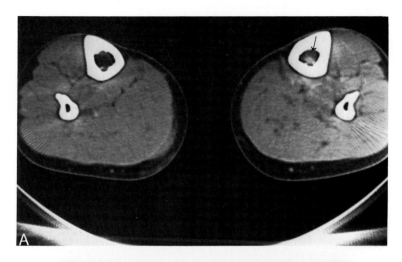

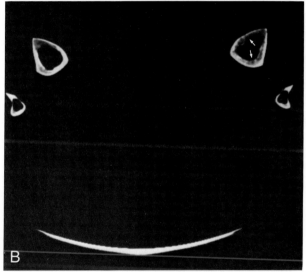

FIG. 5-16. (A) Stress fracture in a 53-year-old woman who enthusiastically embarked on a walking program after treatment for a deep venous thrombosis and presented with a new complaint of calf pain. Conventional radiography showed no definite abnormality. Transaxial CT through the symptomatic level (midcalf) shows asymmetry of the tibial medullary cavities, with increased attenuation of the symptomatic left side (arrow) and a suggestion of subtle tibial thickening laterally and posteriorly. The surrounding soft tissue planes are preserved and symmetrical with the normal side. (B) Widened bone windows (WW 376, WC 1471) at the same level show subtle endosteal reaction and irregularity (arrows). All symptoms resolved with curtailed activity.

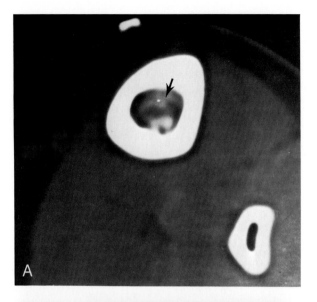

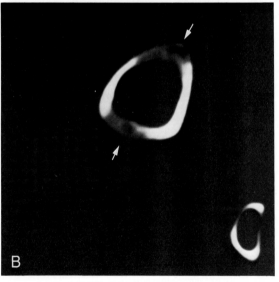

FIG. 5-17. (A) Conventional radiographs of an 8-year-old girl with calf pain for 3 weeks, who denied trauma, showed a subtle, focal permeative lesion of the tibia at the symptomatic level. Transaxial CT at this level (skin marker) showed a mottled increase in medullary cavity attenuation (arrow) and no evidence of soft tissue mass. (B) Wide bone windows (WW 392, WC 1315) revealed permeative lesions of anterior and posterior cortex (arrows). The differential diagnosis included Ewing's sarcoma and stress fracture. On requestioning, the child admitted to 3 months of breakdancing. Resolution of radiographic signs and physical symptoms were noted once this activity was abandoned.

periosteal surfaces.[20] The marrow attenuation, normally fat density (−90 to −120 HU) and symmetric between limbs, may be seen to be increased. Unfortunately, these findings are nonspecific and do not rule out osteomyelitis, Ewing's sarcoma, osteoid osteoma, or other neoplasm. However, in some cases CT may document a distinct fracture line, while failing to uncover, for example, extensive permeative bone destruction or a nidus. The former more definitely rules in stress fracture, while absence of the latter may rule out other entities in the differential. Therefore CT, while potentially nonspecific for stress fracture, can in some cases provide the evidence necessary to allow conservative management of a worrisome lesion, particularly in young patients.[21]

REFERENCES

1. Rockwood CA, Jr., Green DP: Fractures in Adults. JB Lippincott: Philadelphia, 1984

2. Levinsohn EM, Bunnell WP, Yuan HA: Computed tomography in the diagnosis of dislocations of the sternoclavicular joint. Clin Orthop Rel Res 140:12, 1979

3. Destouet JM, Gilula LA, Murchy WA, Sagel SS: Computed tomography of the sternoclavicular joint & sternum. Radiology 138:123, 1981

4. Haynor DR, Shuman WP: Double contrast CT arthography of the glenoid labrum and shoulder girdle. Radiographics 4:411, 1984

5. Whelan MA, Gold RP: Computed tomography of the sacrum: 1. Normal anatomy. AJR 139:1183, 1982

6. Lawson TL, Foley WD, Carrera GF, Berland LL: The sacroiliac joints: anatomic, plain roentgenographic, and computed tomographic analysis. J Comput Assist Tomog 6:307, 1982

7. Vogler JB, III, Broun WH, Helms CA, Genant HK: The normal sacroiliac joint: a CT study of asymptomatic patients. Radiology 151:433, 1984

8. Pennal GF, Tile M, Waddell JP, Garside H: Pelvic disruption: assessment and classification. Clin Orthop Rel Res 151:12, 1980

9. Tile M: Fractures of the acetabulum. Orthop Clin North Am 11(3):481, 1980

10. Gill K, Bucholz RW: The role of computerized tomographic scanning in the evaluation of major pelvic fractures. J Bone Joint Surg 66A(1):34, 1984

11. Fishman ER, Magid D, Brooker AF, Siegelman SS: Fractures of the sacrum and sacroiliac joint—CT MPR/D evaluation. Submitted.

12. Kozin F, Carrera GF, Ryan LM et al: Computed tomography in the diagnosis of sacroiliitis. Arthritis Rheum 24(12):1479, 1981

13. Magid D, Fishman EK, Mandelbaum BR et al: Computed tomography with multiplanar restrucations in the assessment and management of acetabular fractures. J Comput Assist Tomogr (in press).

14. Fishman EK, Magid D, Robertson DD et al: CT/MPR of metallic hip implants. Radiology Sept. 1986 (in press).

15. Weese JL, Rosenthal MS, Gould H: Avoidance of artifacts on computerized tomograms by selection of appropriate surgical clips. Am J Surg 147:684, 1984

16. Geslien GE, Thrall JH, Espinosa JL, Older RA: Early detection of stress fractures using 99m TCc-polyphosphate. Radiology 121(3):683, 1976

17. Collier BD, Johnson RP, Carrera GF et al: Scintigraphic diagnosis of stress-induced incomplete fractures of the proximal tibia. J Trauma 24(2):156, 1984

18. Deveraux MD, Parr GR, Lachmann SM et al: The diagnosis of stress fractures in athletes. JAMA 252(4):531, 1984

19. Greaney RB, Gerber FH, Laughlin RL et al: Distribution and natural history of stress fractures in U.S. Marine recruits. Radiology 146:339, 1983

20. Somer K, Meurman KOA: Computed tomography of stress fractures. J Comput Assist Tomogr 6(1):109, 1982

21. Yousem D, Magid D, Fishman EK et al: CT of stress fracture: potential pitfalls in diagnosis. J Comput Assist Tomogr 10(1):92, 1986

6 The Foot and Ankle

DAVID M. YOUSEM
WILLIAM W. SCOTT, JR.

Because of the extensive overlap of many of the foot bones on standard antero-posterior (AP), lateral, and oblique plain films, CT may be of assistance in evaluating various foot disorders. In particular, the three compartments of the talocalcaneal joint, the transverse tarsal joints, and the tibiotalar joint can be exquisitely defined using CT. In addition, podiatric soft tissue tumors and infectious processes are best evaluated with CT. With its added capacity for multiplanar reconstruction, CT often is more sensitive than linear tomography and more specific than bone scinitigraphy as a second-line study of the foot.

TECHNIQUE

Using the Siemen's DR-3 scanner at 5.2 sec, 449 MAS, and 125 kV, a standard complete examination of the foot and ankle consists of high-resolution 4-mm slices in the coronal and plantar planes. The coronal plane provides optimal orientation for examination of the talocalcaneal joint, and the plantar plane optimally demonstrates talonavicular and calcaneocuboid joints. Similarly, tarsal–metatarsal joints and plantar soft tissue processes are best examined in the plantar plane. While intravenous contrast medium is rarely used for abnormalities confined to the bones, it may be of some use when neoplastic or infectious lesions are suspected and demonstration of their relation to vascular structures is necessary. Finally, the parameters may be adjusted to 2-mm slices, 10-second scans, and various gantry tilts when critical definition of a joint space or lesion margin is required.

Sagittal sections are best reserved for soft tissue plantar lesions or to confirm joint abnormalities suspected on other views. These may be reconstructed from coronal or plantar slices if fine detail is not required.

Guyer et al. have reported that a 22-cut, 5-mm contiguous coronal CT scan, coupled with a 36-cut 1.5-mm contiguous plantar scan would deliver less than one-third (4.3 rads) the radiation to the skin of a 20-cut conventional coronal

113

tomogram study (18 rads).[1] Additionally, examinations in plaster casts could be provided with good quality and without need for orthopedic manipulation.

ANATOMY

A review of the osseous anatomy of the foot demonstrates why CT is of value in diseases of the foot,[2-7] particularly the talus and calcaneus, which constitute the "hindfoot." The talocalcaneal joint consists of three sets of articulating facets divided into two synovial cavities (Fig. 6-1). The posterior, laterally oriented synovial cavity, the subtalar joint, is formed by the respective posterior facets of the talus and calcaneus. The tarsal canal, the talocalcaneal ligament, and, laterally, the tarsal sinus separate the posterior subtalar joint from the medially oriented talocalcaneonavicular joint which contains the middle and anterior facet articulations. The articulation of the sustentaculum tali with the middle talar facet forms the middle talocalcaneal articulation of the talocalcaneonavicular joint. The anterior facets lie anterior and lateral to the middle talocalcaneal joint and are the most difficult to visualize on coronal CT cuts. Although the calcaneus itself does not articulate with the navicular, they do share a common synovial cavity, separate from the calcaneocuboid joint.

The talocalcaneal joint is supported by the deltoid and calcaneonavicular ligaments medially, the calcaneofibular and talofibular ligaments laterally, and the talocalcaneal ligaments circumferentially and inferiorly (Fig. 6-2). Generally, motion at this level consists of inversion and eversion, although minor contributions to abduction–adduction and flexion–extension are provided.

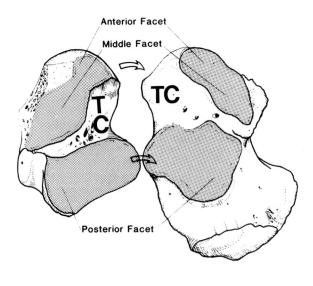

Anterior Facet

Middle Facet

TC

T
C

TC

Posterior Facet

Inferior surface of

TALUS

Superior surface of

CALCANEUS

FIG. 6-1. The talocalcaneal joint is divided into two compartments (shaded grey). The anterior compartment contains the anterior facet and the middle facet. The posterior compartment contains the posterior facet. Between the two compartments the tarsal canal (TC) courses obliquely.

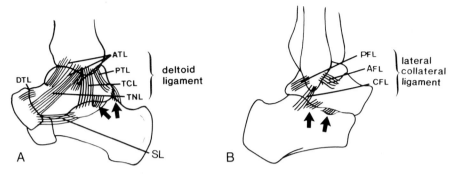

FIG. 6-2. The ligamentous support of the talocalcaneal joint medially (A) is provided by the deltoid ligament, which is separated into the posterior tibiotalar ligament (PTL), the tibiocalcaneal ligament (TCL), the tibionavicular ligament (TNL), and the anterior tibiotalar ligament (ATL). The spring ligament (SL) connects the calcaneus to the navicular medially. Laterally (B), support is provided by the anterior talofibular ligament (AFL), the posterior talofibular ligament (PFL), and the calcaneofibular ligament (CFL), which form the lateral collateral ligament. Further support of the talocalcaneal joint is provided by the medial, lateral, posterior, and interosseous talocalcaneal (small arrows) and dorsal talonavicular ligaments (DTL) that support the talar head and neck.

The transverse tarsal joints (Chopart's joint) consist of the talonavicular and calcaneocuboid joints, which permit gliding motion of the midfoot during inversion and eversion. The navicular, cuboid, and cuneiforms constitute the "midfoot" which lies between Chopart's joint and Lisfranc's tarsal–metatarsal joints (Fig. 6-3).

The tarsal and metatarsal bones distal to Chopart's joint are connected by interosseous ligament forming three sets of arches; one along the cuboid-cuneiform line, one along the metatarsal bases, and one along the metatarsal heads (Fig. 6-4). These provide the ligamentous flexibility for travel on uneven terrain.

The forefoot constitutes the metatarsals and phalanges and their articulations. This area is best examined with plain radiography or plantar CT images.

Coronal CT images of the hindfoot demonstrate the talocalcaneal joint to optimal advantage. The smooth articular surfaces should be unblemished, especially the area of the sustentaculum tali, where early degenerative changes occur. Two critical angles on coronal images were identified by Seltzer: the "heel valgus" angle, which is the angle between the long axes of the tibia and calcaneus, and the "sustentacular angle," the angle of elevation of the sustentaculum tali from the horizontal plane of the ground[4] (Fig. 6-5). This angle is analogous to Ono's "calcaneal inclination angle," which is the angle of the sustentaculum taken from the transverse plane of the ankle mortice, which, when standing, is normally parallel to the ground.[8] The heel valgus angle should be 5.2° ± 1.6°, and the sustentacular/calcaneal inclination angle normally measures 18.3° ± 1.3°. These values should be symmetrical in normal feet. Two other measurements, the medial talar offset, defining the amount of displacement of the anterior head of the talus from the calcaneus and the

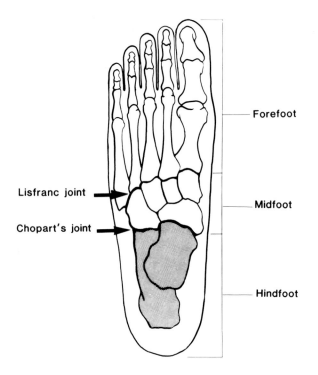

Lisfranc joint

Chopart's joint

Forefoot

Midfoot

Hindfoot

FIG. 6-3. The foot may be divided into the hindfoot, midfoot, and forefoot. Chopart's joint (the "chyma line") separates the hindfoot from midfoot. The Lisfranc tarsometatarsal joint line separates the midfoot from the forefoot. CT's utility is in the evaluation of hindfoot and midfoot disorders.

length of the overhanging portion of the sustentaculum, were determined to be 5.2 ± 1.8 mm and 13.4 ± 0.7 mm, respectively[4] (Fig. 6-6). The sinus tarsi is identified as a fat-filled canal traversing the talocalcaneal joint obliquely.

The normal foot musculature as seen on coronal views may be divided grossly into a dorsal–extensor compartment, a lateral–inversion section, and a plantar–flexor division (Fig. 6-7).

Plantar images of the hindfoot demonstrate to great advantage the talonavicular and the calcaneocuboid joints as well as the plantar talocalcaneal angle; which is the angle of intersection of the AP axes of the talus and calcaneus (normal = 20.1 ± 2.1°)[3] (Fig. 6-8).

While coronal images of the hindfoot are most helpful, plantar images of the midfoot and forefoot are more revealing. These demonstrate the plantar fascia, the deep intrinsic muscles of the foot, the tarsal–metatarsal (Lisfranc), metatarsal–phalangeal, and interphalangeal joints in varying planes of images due to the three sets of arches described earlier (Fig. 6-9). Each tarsal–metatarsal articulation should be smooth without overhanging edges, except the fifth metatarsal base which may project a total of 5 mm lateral to the cuboid. The normal hallux abduction angle should be ≤ 20° on plantar images. Most scans of the forefoot do not pass through the metatarsal–phalangeal plane and these values are therefore better determined on plain films.

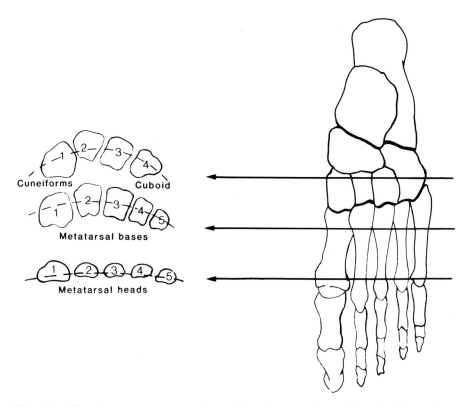

FIG. 6-4. The three transverse arches of the foot run along the cuboid–cuneiform line, the metatarsal bases, and the metatarsal heads.

CONGENITAL DEFORMITIES

The literature supporting CT as the ideal method for demonstrating tarsal coalitions, a cause of rigid flat foot, has accumulated rapidly.[9-12] The most common coalitions, talocalcaneal and calcaneonavicular, are best demonstrated on coronal and plantar views, respectively. Talonavicular and calcaneocuboid coalitions are much rarer, but may also be seen on plantar scans. Talocalcaneal coalitions may be fibrous, cartilaginous, or osseous and generally occur at the medial facet of the anterior talocalcaneonavicular joint, an area poorly visualized on routine plain films (Fig. 6-10). Coronal scans at the region of the sustentaculum tali will nearly always demonstrate bony bridging if it is present at this site. Marked narrowing with or without sclerotic margins suggests fibrous or cartilaginous union in a patient with a spastic flat foot. Secondary findings of talar beaking, degenerative arthritis of the talocalcaneal joint, narrowing of the posterior subtalar joint, and broadening of the lateral aspect of the talus may all be demonstrated with CT and multiplanar reconstructions or on plain films.[9-12]

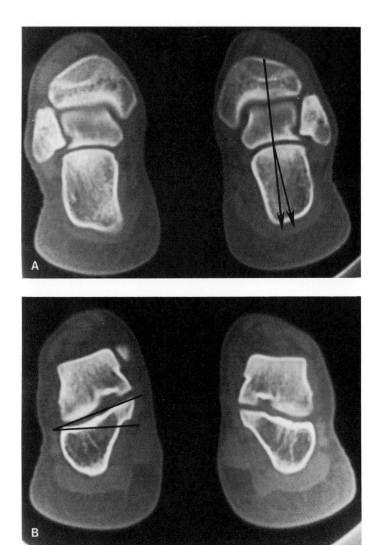

FIG. 6-5. (A) The heel valgus angle is formed by a line through the vertical axis of the tibia and a second line through the vertical axis of the calcaneus (arrows). In normal subjects, the angle is symmetrical and measures 5.2° ± 1.6° (mean ± standard error of the mean). (B) The sustentacular angle is created by drawing a line along the superior edge of the sustentaculum talus at the midsubtalar joint and joining it with a line along the horizontal plane of the ground. This angle is analogous to the calcaneal inclination angle for which the horizontal plane is the superior border of the talus in a standing image. Normal values for these angles are 18.3° ± 1.3°. Both of these angles are obtained using coronal images through the talocalcaneal joint. The reproducibility of the heel valgus angle and the sustentacular angle is variable and these values are not entirely reliable in our experience.

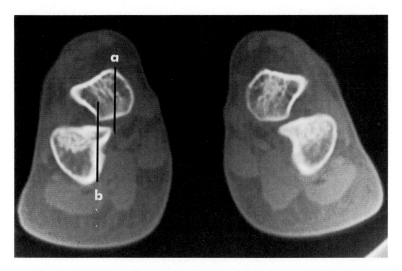

FIG. 6-6.   The medial talar offset is the distance between vertical lines perpendicular to the midpoint of the head of the talus (a) and to the medialmost weight-bearing surface of the calcaneus (b). The distance between these lines defines the amount of displacement of the anterior head of the talus, and usually measures 5.2 ± 1.8 mm. The sustentaculum, which extends medially from the midpoint of the talar head, normally measures 13.4 ± 0.7 mm. Because of the variable widths of the sustentaculum on various coronal slices, these values often vary from scan to scan.

Calcaneonavicular bars are seen on plantar CT images. Because the calcaneus and tarsal navicular do not normally articulate, demonstration of their close proximity, with sclerotic adjacent cortical margins or irregular indistinct borders, may suggest fibrous or cartilaginous union when a bony coalition is not demonstrable[8,10] (Fig. 6-11).

Isolated flat foot deformity or flat feet secondary to tarsal coalitions are suggested by shallow sustentacular angles, low plantar arches demonstrated by early incorporation of anterior forefoot bones on inferior plantar CT scans, and increase of the medial talar offset.[4] Secondary degenerative changes of the talonavicular joint with cortical thickening of the anterior part of the calcaneus (due to altered stress on the foot) also occur. Associated valgus stress will increase the heel valgus angle as well. This diagnosis is more easily made by plain film radiography and CT scanning has limited value unless tarsal coalition is suspected.

Besides tarsal coalitions, other causes of peroneal spastic flatfeet may include rheumatoid arthritis, osteoarthritis, talar osteochondritis, tuberculosis, and trauma. Causes of nonspecific flatfoot deformity diagnosable by CT include vertically oriented talus, degenerative arthritis, unreduced fractures and dislocations. Because both feet are examined easily in the gantry, CT may also detect asymptomatic coalitions in the contralateral foot, reported in as many as 25 percent of cases.[12]

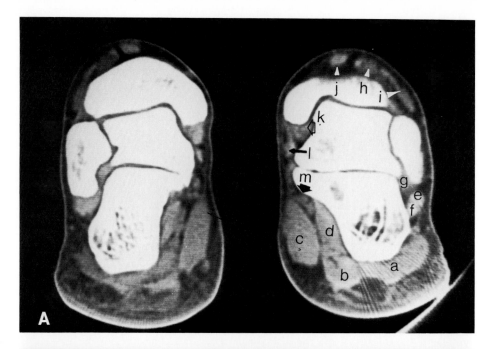

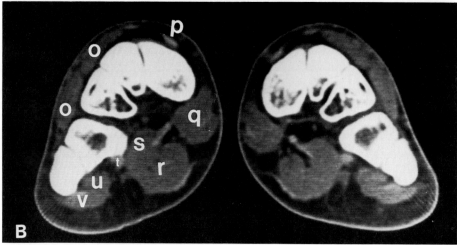

FIG. 6-7. (A) Coronal CT scans using technique to optimize muscle detail demonstrate the posteroinferiorly placed abductor digiti quinti (a), flexor digitorum brevis (b), abductor hallucis (c), and the quadratus plantae (d). Laterally the peroneus brevis tendon (e), peroneus longus tendon (f), and the extensor digitorum brevis tendon (g) are seen. Superoanteriorally one may identify the tendons of the extensor hallucis longus (h), extensor digitorum longus (i), tibialis anterior (j), and the tibialis posterior (k). The flexor digitorum longus tendon (l), and the flexor hallucis longus tendon (m) may be found along the posteromedial aspect of the foot. (B) Coronal CT scan at the level of the metatarsal bases optimized for musculature anatomy. On the dorsum of the feet are the extensor digitorum brevis and longus (o), and the extensor hallucis longus tendon (p). On the plantar aspect one finds, from medial to lateral, the abductor hallucis and flexor hallucis brevis (q), the flexor digitorum brevis (r), the flexor digitorum longus (s), the abductor hallucis tendon (t), the flexor digiti minimi (u), with the abductor digiti minimi (v).

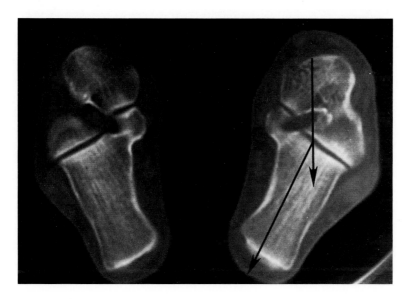

FIG. 6-8.   Lines through the anteroposterior axis of the calcaneus and the talus (arrows) create the plantar talocalcaneal angle, which in normal individuals measures 20.1° ± 2.1°. The inferior portion of the talocalcaneal joint is cut in longitudinal sections in this figure.

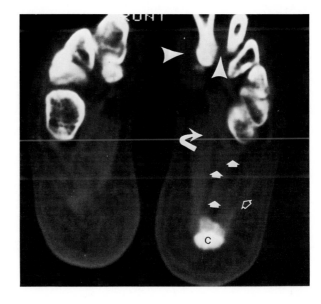

FIG. 6-9.   On this plantar view of the foot the inferior tuberosity of the calcaneus is seen (c) with the slips of the flexor digitorum brevis muscle coursing anteriorly (small white arrows). The flexor hallucis brevis (white arrowheads), abductor hallucis (curved white arrow), and abductor digiti minimi (open white arrow) are visualized. Because of the extensive layering of the flexor musculature and intrinsic foot muscles on plantar images, definable muscle planes are difficult to resolve.

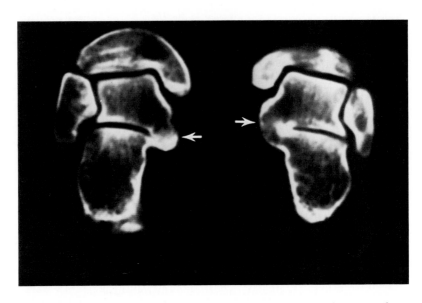

FIG. 6-10. CT scan of a 55-year-old white man with bilateral foot pain for several years' duration and valgus deformity at the ankles demonstrates bony fusion bilaterally at the medial aspect of the talocalcaneal joints; bilateral tarsal coalitions (arrows). A calcaneal spur is visible on the left side.

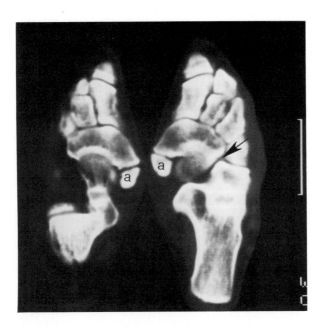

FIG. 6-11. Calcaneonavicular bars are probably best evaluated on oblique AP views of the feet. Plantar CT images may demonstrate bony fusion or, in cases of fibrous or cartilaginous fusion, simple narrowing of the "calcaneonavicular joint" with sclerotic adjacent margins (arrow). This patient has accessory naviculars bilaterally (a).

Grill reported findings of clubfoot deformity on CT scanning including external rotation of the axis of the ankle joint, calcaneocuboid joint deformity,
decrease in the plantar talocalcaneal angle, and increased medial offset of the
navicular on the talus on plantar images.[13] These findings presumably are due
to the continue imbalance of supinator muscles, particularly the tibialis posterior, over the pronator musculature. This supination stress inverts and externally
rotates the foot about the talocalcaneal joint.[13] Persistence of these CT features
in the face of an adequate "shape" to the foot even after surgery suggests
abnormal stresses and alignment of the "treated" clubfoot and may require
secondary operative treatment.[13]

Using frontal linear tomography, Ono reported that in clubfeet narrowing
of the lateral talocalcaneal angle and the sinus tarsi is common, as is hypoplasia
of the sustentaculum tali.[8] The calcaneal inclination angle (sustentacular angle)
at the middle subtalar joint was the most sensitive indicator for equinus and
adductus deformity.[8] This measurement is derived from the horizontal angle
at the middle facet of the talocalcaneal joint to the line of the ankle mortice
(see Fig. 6-5). Mean normal values of 12.7° differed considerably from values
for treated patient's with residual clubfeet, who had values averaging 21.3°.[8]
This measurement reflects the amount of residual supination stress and positioning of the calcaneus from the horizontal (Fig. 6-12).

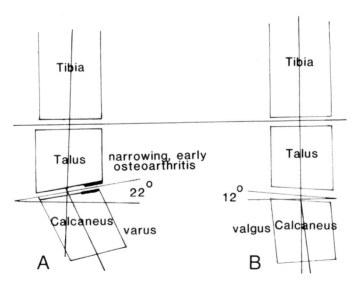

FIG. 6-12.   Ono found that increase in the calcaneal inclination angle (see Fig. 6-5B)
was the most sensitive indication of residual equinovarus deformity on frontal tomography. Other less sensitive findings included increased heel varus deformity and narrowing
of the talocalcaneal joint (A). Compare this with the coronal diagram of a normal
contralateral foot in (B). The abnormal angulation at the talocalcaneal joint may require
further operative treatment. Plantar views may show increased offset of the navicular
from the talus, decrease in the plantar talocalcaneal angle, and calcaneocuboid deformity.

ARTHRITIS

In patients with rheumatoid arthritis 29 percent have subtalar, 39 percent talo-calcaneonavicular, 35 percent tarsometatarsal, and 25 percent calcaneocuboid involvement.[14] All cases with mid- or hindfoot rheumatoid changes showed tarsometatarsal disease as well.[14] Resnick's findings on plain films of soft tissue swelling, cartilage space narrowing, erosions, diffuse osteoporosis, subluxations, and subchondral cysts were demonstrated by CT in six rheumatoid patients by Seltzer et al.[4,14] (Fig. 6-13). The most common foot bone to be involved in rheumatoid arthritis is the calcaneus and its articulations.[14] Increased heel valgus angles, flattened sustentacular angles, and increased medial offsets of the talus may also be seen. While these abnormalities may be better defined by CT than plain films, rheumatoid arthritis remains a clinical or plain film diagnosis. However CT scanning may be useful in planning arthrodesis of affected joints, in analyzing bony impingement or inflammation of muscle tendons, or in determining the degree of cartilaginous loss of the talocalcaneal joint.

Degenerative changes of the hindfoot may be poorly visualized on routine plain films, particularly at its middle facet. In several cases at our institution, CT scanning of a painful foot with normal plain radiographs revealed significant medial compartment cartilage narrowing, spur formation, degenerative cysts, and subarticular sclerosis (Fig. 6-14).

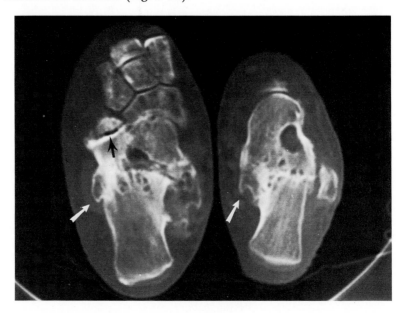

FIG. 6-13. Marked joint space narrowing and areas of fusion of the talocalcaneal joint as well as cyst formation, cortical sclerosis, joint deformity, subluxation at the talonavicular joint, and erosions at the talocalcaneal and talonavicular joints. Spur formation with possible impingement on nearby tendons is present (white arrows). A vacuum cleft at the calcaneocuboid joint is also visible (black arrow).

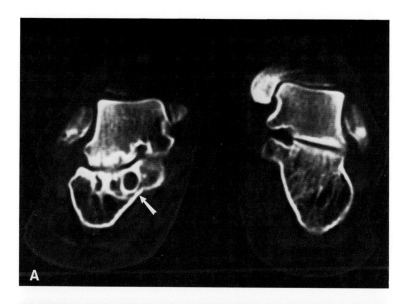

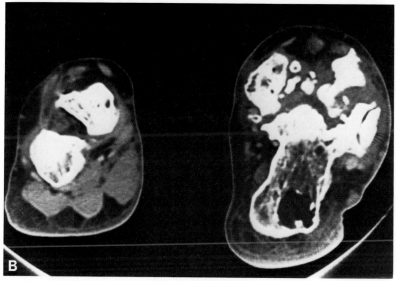

FIG. 6-14. (A) CT scan of a 69-year-old white man with bilateral foot pain of 7 months' duration and relatively normal radiographs of the feet shows moderate sclerosis, narrowing, and cortical irregularity along the lateral aspect of the talocalcaneal joint as well as severe degenerate cyst formation (arrow). These findings are compatible with degenerative arthritis of the hindfoot. (B) The degree of talocalcaneal joint destruction in this case can only be truly appreciated by CT. This was a case of posttraumatic degenerative arthritis.

In a single case of Reiter's syndrome demonstrated by CT, fluffy periostitis, marked narrowing of the talocalcaneal joint, Achilles tendinitis, calcaneal spurs, and a large ankle joint effusion were demonstrated (Fig. 6-15). Reiter's disease affects the foot in greater than 90 percent of cases. The classic arthritic changes of the proximal interphalangeal and metatarsophalangeal joints, Launois's subluxations at these joints, and the presence of calcaneal spurs are best evaluated on plain films.[15] Joint effusions, plantar fasciitis, periarticular erosions, cartilage loss, and subtle periostitis may be better seen by CT however, particularly at the Achilles tendon insertion site on the calcaneus.[15]

Radiodensities suspected of being intrasynovial may be seen with CT, thus negating the need for arthrography. Seltzer reported a case of pigmented villonodular synovitis that demonstrated joint erosion at the articular site of this soft tissue process.[4]

Computed tomographic findings of other foot arthritides such as gout, pseudogout, psoriatic arthritis, and ankylosing spondylitis have not been reported as yet. One would expect findings of chondrocalcinosis, tophi, and joint fusions to be well demonstrated by CT. Similarly, secondary degenerative changes of the hindfoot should be effectively delineated.

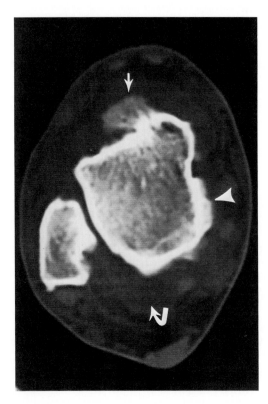

FIG. 6-15. Characteristic findings of joint effusions (curved arrow), spur formation (straight arrow), cortical sclerosis, periostitis (arrowhead), and joint space narrowing are demonstrated in this patient with Reiter's syndrome.

TRAUMA

With compressive injuries to the foot, the sustentacular portion of the calcaneus bears the brunt of the force because of its medial offset from the main calcaneal axis (Fig. 6-16). As such, the talar–sustentacular fracture fragment, with the medial talocalcaneal facet and a variable-sized portion of the posterior facet, is displaced medially and inferiorly. With greater stress, impingement of the lateral fibular malleolus on the lateral calcaneal tuberosity causes comminution of the lateral border of the calcaneus.[15-17] Associated injuries to the calcaneocuboid articulation and the anterior talocalcaneal facet also occur with more severe injury. CT is superior to plain films with hindfoot fractures in determining the degree of comminution of the fractures, the extent of involvement of the three facets of the talocalcaneal joint (especially since 75 percent of calcaneal fractures are intra-articular), the amount of fracture displacement, the location of fracture fragments, and the degree of distortion of Bohler's angle[1,4,17] (Fig. 6-16C). Guyer et al. have shown the value of coronal CT images in determining calcaneal burst fracture fragment impingement on the flexor hallucis longus medially and peroneal tendons laterally.[1] Plantar images will determine talonavicular or calcaneocuboid joint involvement.

While the debate continues concerning whether calcaneal fractures should be treated conservatively or surgically, restoration of the medial wall of the calcaneus is critical in obtaining long-term successful therapy.[15,16,18,19] Displaced intra-articular calcaneal fractures and fractures involving the posterolateral aspect of the posterior facet are treated operatively to reduce the bulge of the laterally displaced calcaneal tuberosity impinging on the peroneal tendons.[15,17,18] Extensive comminution, however, may preclude surgical treatment (Fig. 6-16D). CT is useful in identifying the size, number, and displacement of bone fragments and in determining optimal pin placement or staple positioning for adequate fracture reduction.[17] Whether postoperatively or after manual reduction, CT will demonstrate the extent of any residual displacement or angulation better than plain films. Additionally, late complications of degenerative arthritis of the talocalcaneal joint, facet incongruity, intra-articular bone fragments, osteomyelitis, septic joints, as well as entrapment of muscles and tendons by bony spicules or spurs may be shown.[1,17]

Computed tomography's ability to evaluate both feet in the gantry at the same time is particularly valuable in calcaneal trauma where bilateral fractures have been reported in as many as 7 to 27 percent of cases.[16,21] Stress fractures of the posterior tuberosity of the calcaneus are notoriously difficult to diagnose by plain radiography and CT may assist in clarifying lesions suspected on bone scintigrams.[21] Stress fractures of the calcaneus and metatarsals may be suggested on CT by increased bone marrow density, callus formation, soft tissue swelling, or visualization of a subtle fracture line.[22,23]

Zinman and Reis reported 15 cases of osteochondritis dissecans of the talus evaluated with CT.[24] In four cases, CT demonstrated complete detachment of an osteochondral fragment, thereby necessitating operative treatment, when

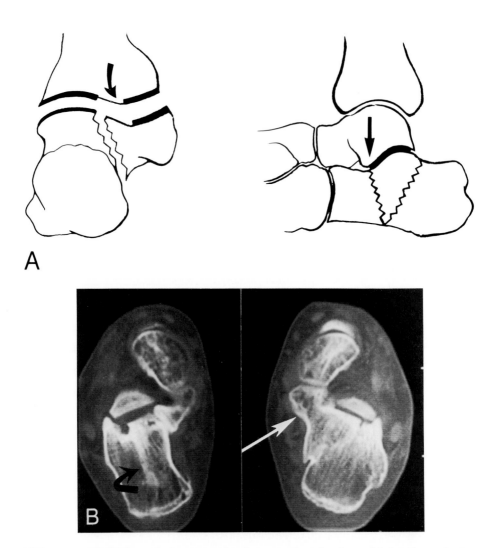

FIG. 6-16.   (A) With vertical compression forces to the talocalcaneal joint, the sustentaculum is separated from the tuberosity, with the former being displaced medially and inferiorly. As the magnitude of the force increases, comminution of the lateral portion of the tuberosity fragment occurs. (B) CT scan demonstrates bilateral healing calcaneal fractures with a triangular fragment of the sustentaculum present on the right (white arrow) and a longitudinal fracture of the calcaneal tuberosity on the left (curved black arrow).

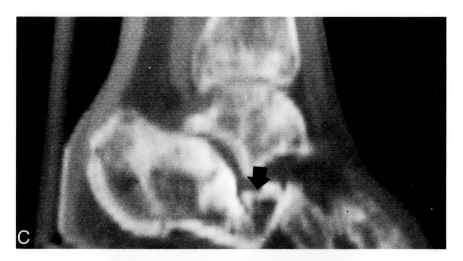

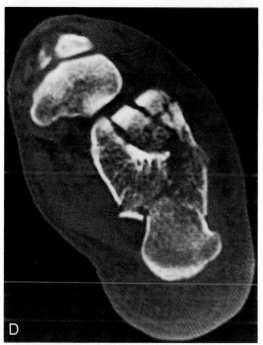

FIG. 6-16. (*continued*)   (C) Sagittal reconstruction of the coronal images of the left foot of the patient in (B) demonstrates decrease in Bohler's angle (normal = 28° to 42°). Note also the depressed fragment of the anterior portion of calcaneus (arrow). (D) CT scan of a comminuted calcaneal fracture involving the talocalcaneal joint aided in surgical evaluation by showing the extreme degree of fragmentation. Nonsurgical management was used.

plain films had suggested only partial fragment detachment and would have dictated conservative therapy.[25] In other cases, CT helped in the planning of optimal surgical management by carefully delineating the extent of the detached superomedial osteochondral fragment of the talus; this was particularly critical in cases where the overlying cartilage appeared entirely normal at surgery.[24]

Another source of plain film confusion in trauma cases is the painful accessory navicular. Although nuclear medicine scanning may suggest that a stress fracture has occurred at the accessory navicular interface, it is nonspecific in determining whether infectious arthritis or neoplastic processes may be present instead.[26] CT may be capable of demonstrating a subtle fracture line or the disruption of the cartilaginous interface.

Avascular necrosis (AVN) of the talus with areas of sclerosis and cyst formation has also been demonstrated by CT. Because many cases of AVN of the talus are associated with fractures, an amount of sclerosis out of proportion to fracture healing as well as deformity of the talar contour suggests posttraumatic AVN (Fig. 6-17). In practice, this determination is probably better evaluated using plain films. Eighty-four percent of type III fractures of the talus, where the body is dislocated from the ankle and subtalar joint, are associated with avascular necrosis.[27] This disrupts the three sources of blood supply to the talus: through the neck, sinus tarsi, and foramina on the medial supply of the body. Type II fractures with subtalar dislocation interrupt blood supply via the neck and sinus tarsi and are associated with a 50 percent incidence of AVN.[27] Type I injuries have minimal talar displacement and a low incidence

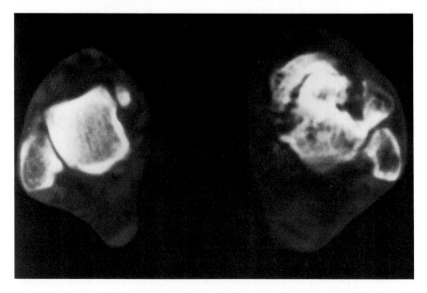

FIG. 6-17. Marked sclerosis of left talus after previous fracture suggests avascular necrosis. With marked comminution of talar fragments, differentiation between callus formation and fracture healing or avascular necrosis becomes difficult. However, the most frequent cause of talar avascular necrosis is trauma.

of AVN. Complications of talar fracture such as malunion, posttraumatic arthritis, and infections may be evaluated efficiently by CT. Avascular necrosis of the talus has also been reported as a complication of pancreatitis.[28]

INFECTION

Ten percent of cases of osteomyelitis occur in the foot.[29] Osteomyelitis may complicate postsurgical treatment of podiatric disorders, diabetic foot ulcers, hematogenous spread of infections, and traumatic injuries to the foot. CT findings in osteomyelitis include an early increase in density of the bone marrow from fat density to soft tissue density, lytic destruction of bone, endosteal and periosteal new bone formation, and soft tissue inflammation[30-32] (Fig. 6-18). Hernandez recently reported the finding of small focal calcific densities inside an inflammatory cavity in bones with osteomyelitis; these may represent sequestra.[33] Visualization of sequestra or intraosseous air (in the medullary cavity) should strongly suggest osteomyelitis.[34]

Soft tissue inflammatory processes in the foot may be identified by detecting air in a soft tissue mass, obliteration of fat planes, and soft tissue swelling. Peripheral contrast medium enhancement of an abscess cavity may also occur. The lack of change in medullary cavity density or bone contours in cellulitis and other soft tissue infections may help to distinguish them from osteomyelitis.

Nonspecific findings of joint effusions, destructive arthritis, and soft tissue swelling may be found with septic arthritides of the foot and ankle.

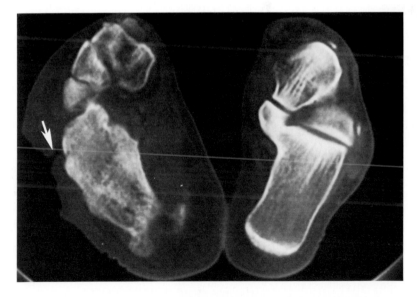

FIG. 6-18. CT scans through the calcaneus in a patient with osteomyelitis demonstrate ill-defined bone destruction and sclerosis in the left calcaneus. Increased soft tissue attenuation due to inflammation is seen laterally, as well as a sinus tract (arrow).

NEOPLASMS

In Dahlin's extensive study of 6,221 cases of bone neoplasms, he reported 35 benign and 38 malignant tumors of the feet.[35] Of the benign tumors, osteoid osteomas, enchondromas, and chondromyxoid fibromas were most common. While plain radiographs should be sufficient to diagnose the latter two, CT may be necessary to identify the margins of an osteoid osteoma as well as its central sclerotic nidus. Two to ten percent of osteoid osteomas occur in the foot, with the talus most frequently affected.[36] Because these occur most frequently in cancellous or subperiosteal bone in the foot, classic reactive sclerosis may be absent, and the diagnosis missed on plain films.[36] Osteoid osteomas may occur subarticularly in the foot where they may induce degenerative changes. The diagnosis may therefore be obscured on plain films by these secondary changes.

Ewing's sarcoma is the most common primary bone malignancy in the foot.[35] Only 3 to 4 percent of all Ewing's sarcomas occur in the foot and of these 50 percent occur in the calcaneus.[37] In contrast to Ewing's sarcomas elsewhere, those in the foot demonstrate less sclerosis and less periosteal reaction, although findings of a lytic lesion, bone expansion, and an extensive adjacent soft tissue

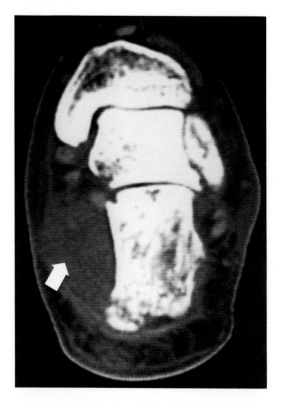

FIG. 6-19. Permeative destruction of the body of the calcaneus on coronal image in a patient with Ewing's sarcoma. Note the large soft tissue component of the tumor medial to the calcaneus, which was not demonstrated on plain film (arrow). The absence of periosteal reaction is not uncommon in Ewing's sarcoma of the feet.

mass continue to be present.[37] This soft tissue component as well as margins of the tumors are best studied using CT (Fig. 6-19).

After Ewing's sarcoma, osteosarcoma, chondrosarcoma, and giant cell tumor are the next most frequent aggressive bony foot neoplasms.[35,38] None of these lesions show contrast enhancement. Again, CT's utility is mostly in demonstrating intramedullary extent of lesions, soft tissue components, skip metastases, relationship to vascular or musculotendinous structures, joint space involvement, and postoperative recurrence of tumors[31,39-42] (Fig. 6-20).

Of nonbony primary malignancies of the foot, fibrosarcoma of the Achilles tendon is most common and would be readily visualized by CT.[35] Other sarcomas are rare in the foot. Benign lipomas, hemangiomas, and neuromas also may be demonstrated and can be distinguished by attenuation and contrast enhancement characteristics. Pseudocapsules of soft tissue tumors may show rim enhancement and help in surgical planning (Fig. 6-21).

In a review of the literature in 1982, Zindrick reported 72 cases of metastases to the feet.[43] These usually arose from primary tumors of the lung, colon, and kidney and occurred most frequently in the tarsals (especially the calcaneus) and metatarsals. While there are no specific characteristics on CT of metastases, the lesions often are purely osteolytic, spare joints, have no periosteal reaction or osteoporosis, and rarely affect the soft tissue.[43,44]

Benign cystic lesions of the foot may be distinguished by CT. While unicameral bone cysts show density readings of less than 20 Hounsfield units (HU), aneurysmal bone cysts (ABC) have soft tissue matrices with densities over 25 HU.[39] The ABC has more expansion, cortical disruption, and trabeculation on CT[45] (Fig. 6-22). Fibrous dysplasia, another bubbly bone lesion, usually has density readings even greater than ABC, over 70 HU, and a fibrous matrix.[46]

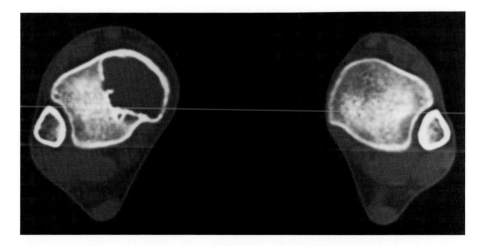

FIG. 6-20.   Giant cell tumor of the distal tibia demonstrating a lytic lesion confined to the bone which extended to the epiphysis. CT scan defined the margins of this tumor for surgical treatment.

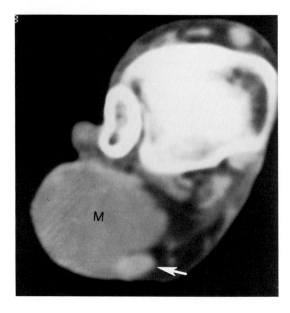

FIG. 6-21. The 4-cm soft tissue mass (M) posterior to the ankle extending laterally and invading several muscle planes was biopsied and proved to be malignant fibrous histiocytoma. The surgical margins for resection were defined by CT scanning. Note the tumor's proximity to the Achilles tendon (arrow).

Periosteal reaction is seen in over 50 percent of all cases of ABC and expansion into soft tissues is seen in 20 percent.[47] These findings are rare in simple cysts or fibrous dysplasia. Thin, peripheral calcification of the ABC's soft tissue component with internal trabeculation is also characteristic of this lesion and easily seen by CT.[48] Dahlin reported five cases of foot ABCs of 134 in the

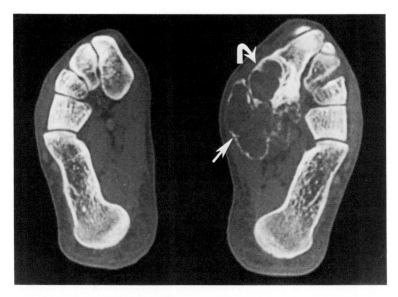

FIG. 6-22. Lytic lesion involving the navicular (straight arrow) and first cuneiform (curved arrow) with marked bony expansion proved to be an aneurysmal bone cyst. Plain films had shown no evidence of involvement of the navicular.

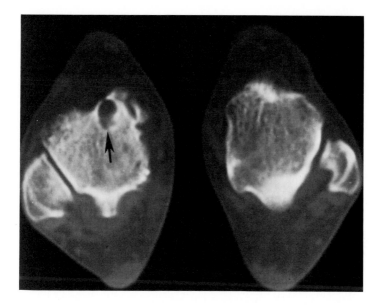

FIG. 6-23.   A 61-year-old man with a 3-year history of right foot pain partially relieved by aspirin was clincially suspected of having an osteoid osteoma. Coronal CT scans of the talus revealed a cystic lesion with a small fluid level (arrow) compatible with the pathologically proven diagnosis of interosseous ganglion cyst.

body.[35] Another cystic lesion, a ganglion cyst, may be identified by its well-defined margins, fluid level, and occasional septation.[49] These lesions may be found in the soft tissue (usually plantar) or intraosseously (Fig. 6-23).

Azouz reported a case of synovial sarcoma that demonstrated calcification on CT, replacement of normal intramedullary fat by tumor, and contrast enhancement.[50] The margins of the tumor were well demarcated by CT, providing a guideline for surgical removal. CT will also demonstrate subtle bony invasion by synovial sarcomas before plain films.[4]

CONCLUSIONS

Reviewing the literature and our experience with computed tomography of the foot leads us to the following conclusions:

1. Its main utility lies in the precise visualization of pathologic change in areas that are typically poorly evaluated by plain films, such as the medial and posterior facets of the talocalcaneal joint and the soft tissues of the foot.

2. Medial tarsal coalitions, sustentacular trauma, soft tissue primary tumors, or soft tissue involvement by primary bone tumors and inflammatory processes will therefore remain reasonable indications for CT evaluation.

3. Computed tomography's utility in studying inflammatory arthritides or osteomyelitis will be limited to the infrequent need for precise preoperative demonstration of affected joint or bone surfaces.

4. Plain film evaluation is sufficient in analyzing most diseases of the forefoot, where the variable planes of the anatomy make CT findings confusing.

ACKNOWLEDGMENT

The authors' thanks go to Judy Baclawski, Diane Robertson, and Elliot K. Fishman for assistance in preparation of the manuscript.

REFERENCES

1. Guyer BH, Levinsohn EM, Fredrickson BE et al: Computed tomography of calcaneal fractures: anatomy, pathology, dosimetry, and clinical relevance. AJR 145:911, 1985
2. Shereff MJ, Johnson KA: Radiographic anatomy of the hindfoot. Clin Orthop Rel Res 177:16, 1983
3. Smith RW, Staple TW: Computerized tomography (CT) scanning technique for the hindfoot. Clin Orthop Rel Res 177:34, 1983
4. Seltzer SE, Weissman BN, Braunstein EM et al: Computed tomography of the hindfoot. J Comput Assist Tomog 8:488, 1984
5. Heger L, Wulff K: Computed tomography of the calcaneus: normal anatomy. AJR 145:123, 1985
6. Feist JH, Mankin HJ: The tarsus. Radiology 79:250, 1962
7. Resnick D: Radiology of the talocalcaneal articulations. Radiology 111:581, 1974
8. Ono K, Hayashi H: Residual deformity of treated congenital club foot. J Bone Joint Surg 56A:1577, 1974
9. Sarno RC, Carter BL, Bankoff MS et al: Computed tomography in tarsal coalition. J Comput Assist Tomogr 8:1155, 1984
10. Deutsch AL, Resnick D, Campbell G: Computed tomography and bone scintigraphy in the evaluation of tarsal coalition. Radiology 144:137, 1982
11. Jones BW, Barranco FT, Fishman EK et al: Imaging techniques in the diagnosis of tarsal coalitions. Adv Orthop Surg 8:264, 1985
12. Beckley DE, Anderson PW, Pedegana LR: The radiology of the subtalar joint with special reference to talo-calcaneal coalition. Clin Radiol 26:333, 1975
13. Grill F: Clubfoot therapy according to Bosch: conservative and operative aspects. Arch Orthop Traum Surg 103:320, 1984
14. Resnick D: Roentgen features of the rheumatoid mid- and hindfoot. J Can Assoc Radiol 27:99, 1976
15. Sholkoff SD, Glickman MG, Steinbach HL: Roentgenology of Reiter's syndrome. Radiology 97:497, 1970
16. Tanke GMH: Fractures of the calcaneus. Acta Chir Scand (suppl 505):1, 1982
17. Soeur R, Remy R: Fractures of the calcaneus with displacement of the thalamic portion. J Bone Joint Surg 57B:413, 1975
18. Heger L, Wulff K, Seddiqi MSA: Computed tomography of calcaneal fractures. AJR 145:131, 1985
19. Burdeaux BD: Reduction of calcaneal fractures by the McReynolds medial approach technique and its experimental basis. Clin Orthop Rel Res 177:87, 1983
20. Omoto H, Sakurada K, Sugi M et al: A new method of manual reduction for intra-articular fracture of the calcaneus. Clin Orthop Rel Res 177:104, 1983

21. Wilson ES, Katz FN: Stress fractures. Radiology 92:481, 1969

22. Yousem DM, Magid D, Fishman EK et al: Computed tomography of stress fractures: pitfalls in diagnosis J Comput Assist Tomogr 10:92, 1986

23. Somer K, Meurman KOA: Computed tomography of stress fractures. J Comput Assist Tomog 6:109, 1982

24. Zinman C, Reis ND: Osteochondritis dissecans of the talus: use of the high resolution computed tomography scanner. Acta Orthop Scand 53:697, 1982

25. Berndt AL, Harty M: Transchondral fractures (osteochondritis dissecans) of the talus. J Bone Joint Surg 41A:988, 1959

26. Lawson JP, Ogden JA, Sella E et al: The painful accessory navicular. Skel Radiol 12:250, 1984

27. Canale ST, Kelly FB, Jr.: Fractures of the neck of the talus. J Bone Joint Surg 60A:143, 1978

28. Baron M, Paltiel H, Lander P: Aseptic necrosis of the talus and calcaneal insufficiency fractures in a patient with pancreatitis, subcutaneous fat necrosis, and arthritis. Arthritis Rheum 27:1309, 1984

29. Antoniou D, Conner AN: Osteomyelitis of the calcaneus and talus. J Bone Joint Surg 56A:338, 1974

30. Kuhn JP, Berger PE: Computed tomographic diagnosis of osteomyelitis. Radiology 130:503, 1979

31. Hermann G, Rose JS: Computed tomography in bone and soft tissue pathology of the extremities. J Comput Assist Tomogr 3:58, 1979

32. Hald JK Jr., Sudmann E: Acute hematogenous osteomyelitis. Acta Radiol 23:55, 1982

33. Hernandez RJ: Visualization of small sequestra by computerized tomography. Pediatr Radiol 15:238, 1985

34. Ram PC, Martinez S, Korobkin M et al: CT detection of intraosseous gas: a new sign of osteomyelitis. AJR 137:721, 1981

35. Dahlin DC: Bone Tumors, 3rd ed. Charles C. Thomas, Springfield, Illinois, 1978

36. Shereff MJ, Cullivan WT, Johnson KA: Osteoid-osteoma of the foot. J Bone Joint Surg 65A:638, 1983

37. Reinus WR, Gilula LA, Shirley SK et al: Radiographic appearance of Ewing sarcoma of the hands and feet. AJR 144:331, 1985

38. Coley BL, Higinbotham NL: Tumors primary in the bones of the hand and feet. Surgery 5:112, 1939

39. deSantos LA, Goldstein HM, Murray JA et al: Computed tomography in the evaluation of musculoskeletal neoplasms. Radiology 128:89, 1978

40. deSantos LA, Bernardino ME, Murray JA: Computed tomography in the evaluation of osteosarcoma: experience with 25 cases. AJR 132:535, 1979

41. Berger PE, Kuhn JP: Computed tomography of tumors of the musculoskeletal system in children. Radiology 127:171, 1978

42. Heelan RT, Watson RC, Smith J: Computed tomography of lower extremity tumors. AJR 132:933, 1979

43. Zindrick MR, Young MP, Daley RJ et al: Metastatic tumors of the foot. Clin Orthop Rel Res 170:219, 1982

44. Mulvey RB: Peripheral bone metastases. AJR 91:155, 1964

45. Hertzanu Y, Mendelsohn DB, Gottschalk F: Aneurysmal bone cyst of the calcaneus. Radiology 151:51, 1984

46. Blumberg ML: CT of iliac unicameral bone cysts. AJR 136:1231, 1981

47. Bonakdarpour A, Levy WM, Aegerter E: Primary and secondary aneurysmal bone cyst: a radiologic study of 75 cases. Radiology 126:75, 1978

48. Wang AM, Lipson SJ, Haykal HA et al: Computed tomography of aneurysmal bone cyst of the L₁ vertebral body. J Comput Assist Tomogr 8:1186, 1984

49. Engdahl DE, Kaufman RA, Hopson CN: Computed tomography in the diagnosis of a rare plantar ganglion cyst in a child. J Bone Joint Surg 65-A:1348, 1983

50. Azouz EM, Vickar DB, Brown KLB: Computed tomography of synovial sarcoma of the foot. J Can Assoc Radiol 35:85, 1984

7 The Shoulder

CHARLES S. RESNIK

Numerous abnormalities of the glenohumeral joint and surrounding structures are ideally depicted by CT. Pathologic alterations of the soft tissues may be identified in neuromuscular diseases as well as various neoplastic and infiltrative disorders. Bony alterations in patients with instability of the shoulder often are more easily evaluated by CT than by plain radiography or conventional tomography. Capsular and glenoid labral abnormalities are best defined by CT following instillation of contrast into the glenohumeral joint. This chapter reviews the normal anatomy of the glenohumeral joint and illustrates the role of CT in diagnosing abnormalities of the joint and surrounding structures.

NORMAL ANATOMY

The anatomy of individual muscles surrounding the glenohumeral joint is often well demonstrated by CT.[1] The supraspinatus and infraspinatus may be identified immediately adjacent to the posterior surface of the scapula. The teres major and teres minor are also located posteriorly and inferiorly, while the subscapularis is seen directly anterior to the scapula. The triceps brachii can be seen just posterior to the proximal humerus, and the biceps brachii lies immediately anterior to this bony structure. The deltoid is located more superficially surrounding the lateral aspect of the shoulder. Additional muscles visualized include the pectoral and paraspinal groups.

Articular anatomy of the glenohumeral joint is demonstrated best by CT following intra-articular contrast injection, although noncontrast CT displays osseous anatomy equally well. The method used to perform computed arthrotomography (CAT) varies only slightly in reported series.[2-7] One to 4 milliliters of iodinated contrast material and approximately 10 cc room air are injected by routine arthrographic technique. CT examination is then carried out with the patient in the standard supine position with the shoulder in a neutral or slightly internally rotated orientation. Five to 15 contiguous or overlapping sections 3- to 5-mm thick are obtained beginning at the level of the acromion process and extending inferiorly through the entire glenoid labrum. Scans with the shoulder in external rotation may be added for better visualization of posterior articular structures.[2,6]

On a transaxial image, the central third of the humeral head articular surface normally articulates with the central third of the glenoid fossa.[8] The articular surface of the head is covered by hyaline cartilage and describes a smooth convex arc (Fig. 7-1). The humeral head appears essentially round on superior scans at the level of the coracoid process (Fig. 7-2). More inferiorly, this rounded contour is altered by the outward projections of the greater and lesser tuberosities. Between these latter two structures lies the groove for the tendon of the long head of the biceps muscle; this groove varies greatly in depth and configuration (Fig. 7-1). The normal humeral neck may show loss of definition and spiculation of cortex in some instances.[9]

The articular surface of the glenoid fossa is slightly concave and is covered by hyaline cartilage that is normally thinner at the center than at the periphery.[2,6] The cross-sectional appearance of the posterior margin of the fossa is larger and more rounded than the anterior margin, which has a normal pointed configuration (Fig. 7-1). The glenoid surface is slightly retroverted superiorly but gradually twists to become mildly anteverted more inferiorly. The body of the scapula remains virtually perpendicular to the glenoid fossa at all levels.[8]

The glenoid labrum is a fibrous and fibrocartilaginous structure shaped like a washer and firmly attached circumferentially to the edge of the glenoid fossa. The base of the labrum abuts the articular cartilage of the glenoid, but incomplete attachment sometimes allows for slight, normal separation of these two structures[2,6] (Fig. 7-3). In cross-section, the labrum is essentially triangular in shape. The apex of the anterior labrum often appears pointed, although the usual configuration is more smooth and rounded (Figs. 7-1, 7-4). The anterior and posterior portions are usually equal in size.

The fibrous capsule of the glenohumeral joint is often quite loose and redundant. It is continuous with the capsular border of the labrum and the immediately adjacent bone posteriorly and inferiorly, while its relationship to the scapula anteriorly and superiorly is less precise.[2,6] There are two constant recesses of variable size in the capsule; the subscapular recess lies between the subscapularis muscle and the scapula, and the axillary recess projects between the scapula and the neck of the humerus. The anterior portion of the capsule thickens to form the superior, middle, and inferior glenohumeral ligaments, which course from the anterior margin of the glenoid fossa to the proximal humerus. These structures are variable in configuration and degree of development; the superior ligament is the one most commonly identified[2] (Fig. 7-5). The subscapular recess communicates with the glenohumeral joint through an opening between the superior and middle glenohumeral ligaments, with a large recess corresponding to a well-developed middle ligament and a small recess corresponding to a poorly developed one. The stability of the anterior capsular mechanism is related to the strength of the glenohumeral ligaments.[2]

Important tendons related to the glenohumeral joint include those of the rotator cuff, the long head of the triceps muscle, and the long head of the

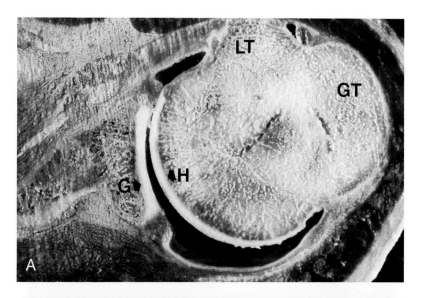

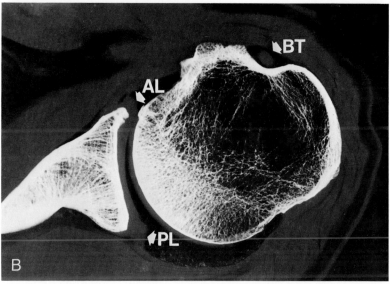

Fig. 7–1. Photograph (A) and radiograph (B) of a transverse section through a cadaveric shoulder following intra-articular injection of air. Structures identified are the humeral articular cartilage (H), glenoid articular cartilage (G), greater tuberosity (GT), lesser tuberosity (LT), biceps tendon and air-filled sheath within the bicipital groove (BT), anterior glenoid labrum (AL), and posterior glenoid labrum (PL). (Resnik CS, Deutsch AL, Resnick D et al: Arthrotomography of the shoulder. RadioGraphics 4:963, 1984.)

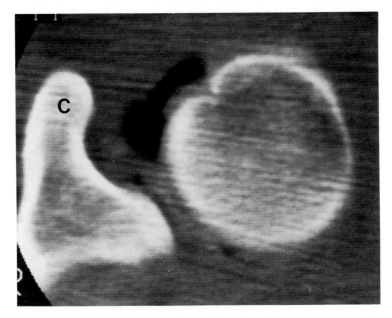

Fig. 7–2. CAT section at the level of the coracoid process (C) showing the normal round appearance of the humeral head. (Resnik CS, Deutsch AL, Resnick D et al: Arthrotomography of the shoulder. RadioGraphics 4:963, 1984.)

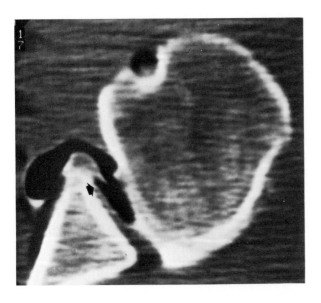

Fig. 7–3. Normal separation of the base of the anterior glenoid labrum from the glenoid articular cartilage with air between these two structures (arrow). (Resnik CS, Deutsch AL, Resnick D et al: Arthrotomography of the shoulder. Radiographics 4:963, 1984.)

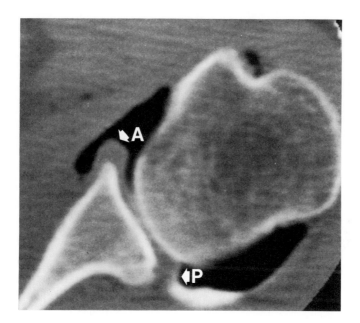

Fig. 7–4. Normal smoothly rounded anterior (A) and posterior (P) glenoid labrum. (Resnik CS, Deutsch AL, Resnick D et al: Arthrotomography of the shoulder. Radio-Graphics 4:963, 1984.)

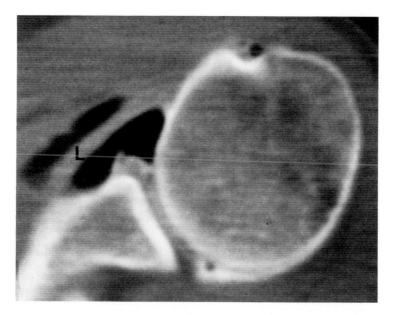

Fig. 7–5. Air outlining a prominent glenohumeral ligament (L).

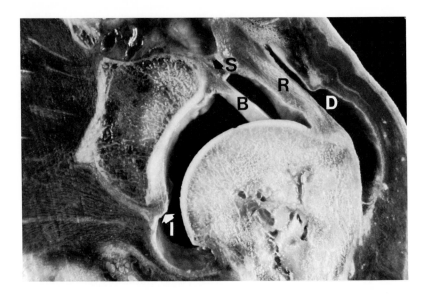

Fig. 7–6. Coronal section through a cadaveric shoulder following intra-articular injection of air showing the superior glenoid labrum (S), inferior glenoid labrum (I), biceps tendon traversing the joint (B), and rotator cuff (R) separating the glenohumeral joint from the air filled subacromial–subdeltoid bursa (D). (Resnik CS, Deutsch AL, Resnick D et al: Arthrotomography of the shoulder. RadioGraphics 4:963, 1984.)

biceps muscle. The latter arises from the superior portion of the glenoid labrum, traverses the joint in a slightly cephalad direction, courses inferiorly within the bicipital groove, and exits the articulation in front of the humeral neck (Figs. 7-1, 7-6). The rotator cuff consists of the supraspinatus, infraspinatus, teres minor, and subscapularis tendons, and separates the glenohumeral joint from the subacromial–subdeltoid bursa (Fig. 7-6). The joint capsule is reinforced superiorly by the supraspinatus, posteriorly by the infraspinatus and teres minor, anteriorly by the subscapularis, and inferiorly by the triceps.

ABNORMAL FINDINGS ON CT

Abnormalities of soft tissue structures surrounding the glenohumeral joint may be demonstrated by CT. Generalized pathologic changes in the musculature can be seen in patients with neuromuscular diseases. Density measurements may be altered, and focal or diffuse atrophy can be easily evaluated.[10] Focal soft tissue masses secondary to neoplastic or infiltrative disorders are also evaluated well by CT.[11] As in other parts of the body, relationships to adjacent vascular structures and invasion of bone are readily identified.[12]

Computed tomography without arthrography can be used to evaluate bony abnormalities accompanying instability or dislocation of the glenohumeral joint. Actual subluxation or dislocation is easily diagnosed if the central third of the humeral articular surface does not project within the central third of the

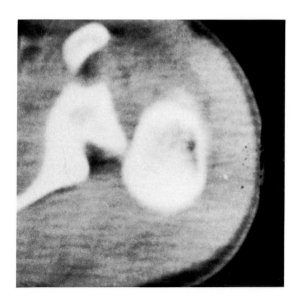

Fig. 7–7. Computed tomographic section showing posterior dislocation of the humeral head.

glenoid fossa[8] (Fig. 7-7). Deformity of the humeral head following anterior glenohumeral dislocation, known as the Hill–Sachs lesion, is represented by flattening or depression of its posterolateral aspect. This is usually evident on routine radiographic examination with the humerus held in internal rotation, but numerous special views have been developed to identify this bony defect in more subtle cases. CT has proven to be an ideal modality for this demonstration[8,13] (see Fig. 7-15). Impaction of the medial aspect of the humeral head secondary to posterior glenohumeral dislocation is also well demonstrated (Fig. 7-8).

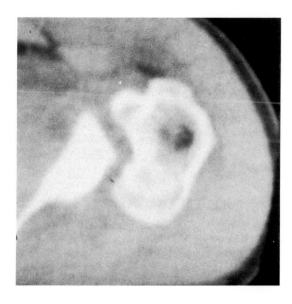

Fig. 7–8. Impaction fracture of the medial humeral head secondary to posterior glenohumeral dislocation.

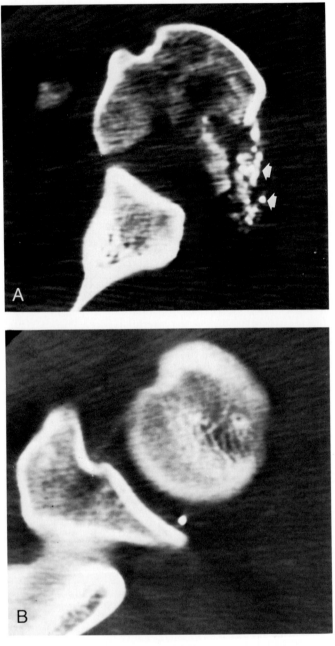

Fig. 7–9. (A) Extensive destruction of the articular surface of the humeral head secondary to gunshot wound. Multiple metal densities are present adjacent to the disrupted lateral cortex (arrows). (B) Section at a higher level showing a single intra-articular metal fragment or pellet.

Associated deformity of the bony glenoid and other miscellaneous disorders are also readily identified by CT. The Bankart lesion, characterized by fracture of the anterior rim of the glenoid following anterior dislocation, may be accompanied by abnormal angulation of the articular surface or more extensive scapular fracture.[8] Postoperative evaluation of osteochondral grafts performed to promote bony healing following fracture is more easily carried out by CT than by plain film radiography.[14] Intra-articular osseous bodies can also be localized more accurately by CT.[8,15] The extent of traumatic damage to bony structures is ideally depicted (Fig. 7-9), as is bony involvement with neoplastic processes (Fig. 7-10).[16] Finally, incidental abnormalities, such as calcific tendinitis or changes of degenerative joint disease, may be observed.

ABNORMAL FINDINGS ON COMPUTED ARTHROTOMOGRAPHY

Computed arthrotomography (CAT) is one of two accurate methods to evaluate the glenoid labrum in patients with instability of the shoulder. Although labral pathologic change may be exquisitely demonstrated by conventional tomography following routine arthrography, CAT has been shown to be slightly more accurate, is better tolerated by patients because of the simplicity of positioning, requires less technical expertise to perform, and produces less patient radiation.[2,6] In addition, CAT is a more comprehensive examination of the

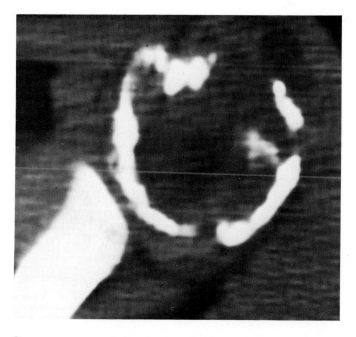

Fig. 7–10. Osteosarcoma involving the humeral head with multiple sites of cortical breakthrough.

glenohumeral joint, allowing better evaluation of articular and surrounding structures.

The abnormality most frequently encountered during CAT is disruption of the normal integrity of the anterior glenoid labrum. Iodinated contrast material or air extending into the substance of the labrum is diagnostic of a tear (Fig. 7-11). Other abnormalities include blunting, thinning, fraying, or imbibition of contrast material along the free margin (Fig. 7-12). Absence of visualization of the labrum is indicative of avulsion or detachment. Similar findings may be observed much less frequently in the posterior aspect of the labrum (Fig. 7-13).

The sensitivity of CAT in the detection of labral abnormalities has been excellent. In the largest reported series of patients undergoing this procedure, Deutsch and co-workers described an overall sensitivity of 96 percent; the sensitivity of detecting anterior labral pathologic change was 100 percent.[2] Other smaller series have also indicated an accuracy of 100 percent.[4,7]

Bony abnormalities involving the glenoid or the humeral head can be identified by CAT just as they can by CT without arthrography. It is important to include appropriate bone window settings to avoid overlooking subtle cortical pathologic conditions. Fractures of the bony glenoid rim are usually associated with disruption of the labrum (Fig. 7-14). A Hill-Sachs lesion of the humeral head is easily identified as flattening or depression of the posterolateral aspect.

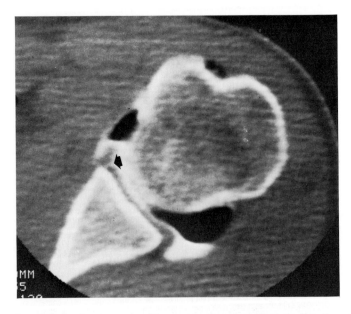

Fig. 7–11. Computed arthrotomographic section showing a linear collection of iodinated contrast within the anterior glenoid labrum, indicative of a small tear (arrow). (Resnik CS, Deutsch AL, Resnick D et al: Arthrotomography of the shoulder. RadioGraphics 4:963, 1984.)

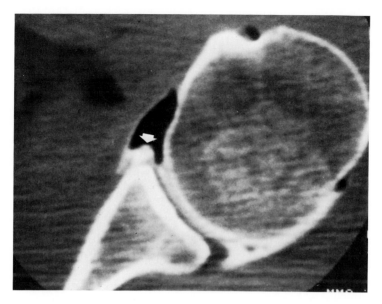

Fig. 7–12. Large collection of iodinated contrast within the anterior glenoid labrum, indicative of a tear (arrow). (Resnik CS, Deutsch AL, Resnick D et al: Arthrotomography of the shoulder. RadioGraphics 4:963, 1984.)

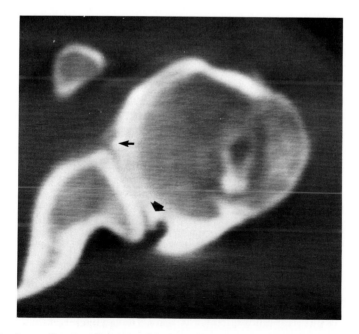

Fig. 7–13. Large linear collection of iodinated contrast within the posterior glenoid labrum, indicative of a tear (large arrow). Also note small tear of the anterior labrum (small arrow).

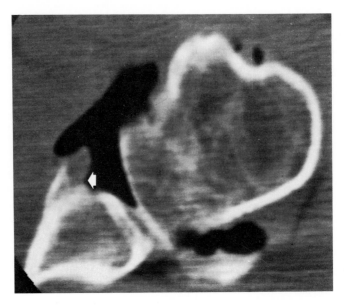

Fig. 7–14. Fracture of the anterior bony glenoid with associated disruption of the labrum (arrow). (Resnik CS, Deutsch AL, Resnick D et al: Arthrotomography of the shoulder. RadioGraphics 4:963, 1984.)

This is best observed at the level of the coracoid process where the head should normally be completely round (Fig. 7-15). Care must be taken not to misinterpret the normal concavity of the junction between articular cartilage and bone along the neck of the humerus at the origin of the greater tuberosity as an abnormal bony defect (Fig. 7-1).

Evaluation of abnormalities of the glenohumeral joint capsule has been reported to be very accurate by several authors.[3-5,7] An increase in size of the anterior joint space may be associated with capsular stretching and stripping of the capsule from its attachment to the anterior glenoid. Intra-articular septa or adhesions may also be demonstrated. However, one large series indicates that there are limitations in making an accurate diagnosis of capsular pathologic change.[2] The normal appearance of the capsule shows a large amount of variability, and distention of the anterior portion of the joint is dependent upon the amount of air injected as well as the position of the shoulder. Deutsch and co-workers noted that all patients with surgically demonstrated capsular abnormalities had coexistent labral abnormalities evident on CAT. They concluded that the criteria used by others may lead to an increased rate of false-positive diagnosis without any increase in sensitivity.[2] Nonetheless, ballooning of the capsule apparently does occur in the absence of other abnormalities; the significance of this finding remains somewhat controversial.

Abnormalities of the biceps tendon or the bicipital groove are ideally demonstrated by CAT. Rupture of the tendon results in its nonvisualization within the normal air-filled sheath (Fig. 7–16). Posttraumatic adhesions or postsurgical

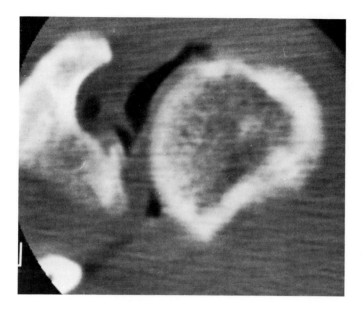

Fig. 7–15. Computed arthrotomographic section showing a Hill-Sachs lesion along the posterolateral aspect of the humeral head (compare to Fig. 7–2). (Resnik CS, Deutsch AL, Resnick D et al: Arthrotomography of the shoulder. RadioGraphics 4:963, 1984.)

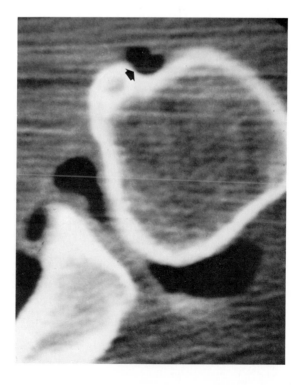

Fig. 7–16. Absence of the biceps tendon within the air-filled sheath secondary to tendon rupture and retraction (arrow).

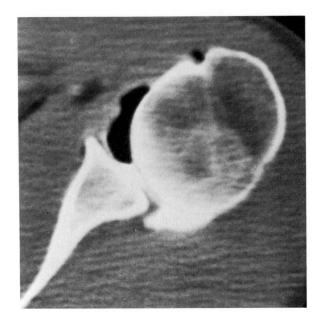

Fig. 7–17. Posterior sub-luxation of the humeral head despite a normal appearing posterior glenoid labrum. (Resnik CS, Deutsch AL, Resnick D et al: Arthrotomography of the shoulder. RadioGraphics 4:963, 1984.)

tenodesis may result in an inability to fill the sheath.[2] CAT would appear to be the imaging modality of choice to diagnose positional abnormalities of the biceps tendon, such as medial dislocation or subluxation. Associated structural deformity of the bicipital groove can be evaluated simultaneously.

Other abnormalities involving glenohumeral joint structures may be observed by CAT. Subluxation or dislocation of the joint is readily apparent as it is on CT without arthrography (Fig. 7–17). Similarly, disorders of osseous development of the glenoid or humerus can be ideally evaluated.[2] Thinning of the

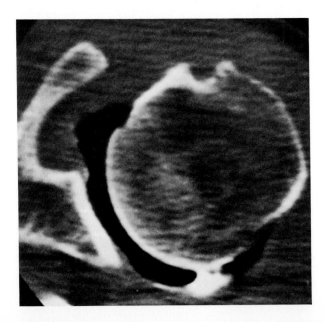

Fig. 7–18. Thinning of the central portion of the glenoid articular cartilage. (Resnik CS, Deutsch AL, Resnick D et al: Arthrotomography of the shoulder. RadioGraphics 4:963, 1984.)

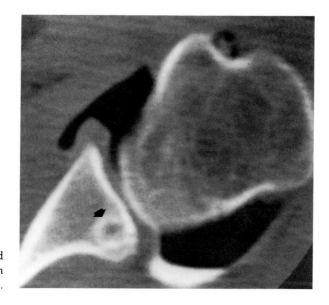

Fig. 7–19. Well-defined subchondral cyst within the bony glenoid (arrow).

articular cartilage of the glenoid or subchondral bone cysts may be demonstrated (Figs. 7–18, 7–19). Loose osteocartilaginous bodies can be specifically localized as intra-articular (Fig. 7–20). Finally, disruption of the rotator cuff can be documented by CAT, although this diagnosis is more easily made during routine arthrography.[3]

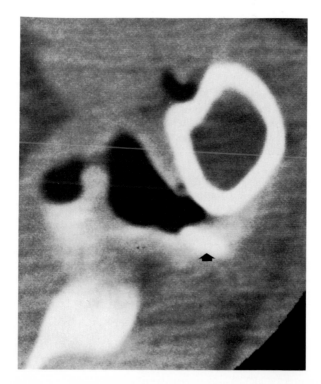

Fig. 7–20. Intra-articular osseous loose body (arrow). (Resnik CS, Deutsch AL, Resnick D et al: Arthrotomography of the shoulder. RadioGraphics 4:963, 1984.)

SUMMARY

Computed tomography is an ideal imaging modality for the evaluation of bony and soft tissue structures of the shoulder. CT performed following routine arthrography can demonstrate intra-articular anatomy exquisitely. This is particularly important in the evaluation of patients with instability of the shoulder, since the glenoid labrum cannot be visualized as easily by any other means. Accurate identification of posttraumatic deformities can aid the orthopedic surgeon in determining the most efficacious method of therapy.

REFERENCES

1. Bulcke JA, Termote J-L, Palmers Y, Crolla D: Computed tomography of the human skeletal muscular system. Neuroradiology 17:127, 1979
2. Deutsch AL, Resnick D, Mink JH et al: Computed and conventional arthrotomography of the glenohumeral joint: normal anatomy and clinical experience. Radiology 153:603, 1984
3. Haynor DR, Shuman WP: Double contrast CT arthrography of the glenoid labrum and shoulder girdle. RadioGraphics 4:411, 1984
4. Kinnard P, Gordon D, Levesque RY, Bergeron D: Computerized arthrotomography in recurring shoulder dislocations and subluxations. Can J Surg 27:487, 1984
5. Kinnard P, Tricoire J-L, Levesque RY, Bergeron D: Assessment of the unstable shoulder by computed arthrography. A preliminary report. Am J Sports Med 11:157, 1983
6. Resnik CS, Deutsch AL, Resnick D et al: Arthrotomography of the shoulder. RadioGraphics 4:963, 1984
7. Shuman WP, Kilcoyne RF, Matsen FA et al: Double-contrast computed tomography of the glenoid labrum. AJR 141:581, 1983
8. Seltzer SE, Weissman BN: CT findings in normal and dislocating shoulders. J Can Assoc Radiol 36:41, 1985
9. Paling MR: The computed tomography of normal long bone anatomy and its simulation of disease. Comput Tomogr 5:201, 1981
10. Termote J-L, Baert A, Crolla D et al: Computed tomography of the normal and pathologic muscular system. Radiology 137:439, 1980
11. Hermann G, Yeh H-C, Schwartz I: Computed tomography of soft-tissue lesions of the extremities, pelvic and shoulder girdles: sonographic and pathological correlations. Clin Radiol 35:193, 1984
12. Lloyd TV, Paul DJ: Erosion of the scapula by a benign lipoma: computed tomography diagnosis. J Comput Assist Tomogr 3:679, 1979
13. Danzig L, Resnick D, Greenway G: Evaluation of unstable shoulders by computed tomography. A preliminary study. Am J Sports Med 10:138, 1982
14. Roffman M, Barmeir E, Dubowitz B et al: The role of computed tomography in the management of osteochondral grafts. Clin Orthop Rel Res 166:112, 1982
15. Gould R, Rosenfield AT, Friedlaender GE: Loose body within the glenohumeral joint in recurrent anterior dislocation: CT demonstration. J Comput Assist Tomogr 9:404, 1985
16. DeSmet AA, Levine E, Neff JR: Tumor involvement of peripheral joints other than the knee: arthrographic evaluation. Radiology 156:597, 1985

8 Measurement of Bone Mineral for Early Detection of Osteoporosis

GOPALA U. RAO
WILLIAM W. SCOTT, JR.
THOMAS J. BECK

WHAT IS OSTEOPOROSIS?

Osteoporosis is a skeletal condition characterized by considerable diminution of bone mass, although the bone that is present may still be adequately mineralized. The thickness and the number of trabeculae are decreased and the cortex is thinned. After reaching skeletal maturity at 30 to 35 years of age, all humans begin to lose bone mineral. The rate of loss may vary between individuals and the amount of mineral present at skeletal maturity may differ. At the present time there is no absolute definition for osteoporosis. The amount of bone mineral loss at which a person is defined as osteoporotic is arbitrary. Some definitions that might be useful include the following: (1) a level of bone mineral lower than that present in young adults at the low end of the normal range, (2) the occurrence of osteoporosis-related fractures, or (3) a level of bone mineral corresponding to that at which osteoporosis-related fractures are likely to occur.

A few facts about osteoporosis will give the reader some perspective as to the important problems involved with this disorder and the segment of the population most likely to suffer from osteoporosis.

Osteoporosis can be divided into two broad categories: senile and postmenopausal. After the age of 30 to 40 years, everyone begins to lose bone mineral. Those who have less mineral than normals at any given age, either because they have lost the mineral more rapidly or had less of it to begin with at maturity, constitute the population with senile osteoporosis. Postmenopausal osteoporosis refers to the relatively rapid mineral loss that occurs in certain women after the menopause. This form of osteoporosis appears to be related to the loss of estrogen at the time of menopause, as treatment with exogenous estrogen can frequently slow or halt the process.[1] There are data to indicate that changes in cancellous bone, a major component of the vertebral body, may be especially rapid compared with cortical bone changes. These changes can be identified by modern techniques.[2] At skeletal naturity, women have less bone mineral than men and whites less than blacks.[3] Women lose bone mineral more rapidly than men. Elderly white women are thus the most susceptible candidates for the onset of osteoporosis. Lack of physical activity, cigarette smoking, lower than average body weight, poor dietary intake of calcium, high protein intake, excessive alcohol use, and exercise sufficiently strenuous to cause amenorrhea, are also believed to play a role in the development of osteoporosis. Superimposed treatment with steroid medications, oophorectomy, or the premature onset of menopause constitute additional risk factors.[4-6]

CLINICAL SIGNIFICANCE

The so-called osteoporosis-related fracture syndromes are the cause of the morbidity and mortality associated with this disorder. Vertebral compression fractures are generally seen in white women over the age of 45 with an average annual fracture rate of 7 percent per year in osteoporotic patients.[7] They commonly occur at the T8 to L2 level and usually are precipitated by routine daily activities. Some are asymptomatic, but they may result in considerable pain and discomfort. A patient eventually becomes kyphotic and loses height. Ninety-six percent of such patients will demonstrate six or more fractures over a period of 10 years.[8] The same group of patients is also subject to fractures of the distal radius. The incidence of these increases dramatically in white women over the age of 40.[7] The increased frequency of falls in elderly patients may be a contributing factor in these injuries.[9,10] However, these fractures usually heal well with little residual disability. Fractures of the neck and the intertrochanteric region of the femur are a third important fracture type. A typical patient is a white woman in her late 70s. These fractures frequently occur following mild trauma, such as a fall on level ground,[7] and entail significant morbidity and mortality. The average hospital stay is approximately 20 days. There is an approximately 30 percent complication rate, including displacement, nonunion, aseptic necrosis, and prosthetic loosening. Mortality rate[11] within 1 year due to the fracture is about 20 percent.

CONDITIONS CONFUSED WITH OSTEOPOROSIS

Anyone dealing with the detection of osteoporosis should keep in mind that slightly less than 1 percent of the time some other underlying disorder can mimic senile or postmenopausal osteoporosis. When a patient presents with a fracture complicating what appears to be osteoporosis, the possiblity of some other condition, such as osteomalacia, hyperparathyroidism, multiple myeloma, and metastases should be considered. Some of these will have diagnostic findings on plain film examination. Pseudofractures may suggest osteomalacia. Focal lytic lesions suggest myeloma or metastases. Subperiosteal bone resorption is rather specific for hyperparathyroidism. The diagnosis of osteomalacia, if suspected, usually requires bone biopsy for confirmation. Serum protein electrophoresis confirms the diagnosis of multiple myeloma. Biopsy of a bone lesion or identification and biopsy of a primary malignancy is necessary to confirm bony metastases when they are suspected on skeletal films.

WHAT CAN BE DONE ABOUT OSTEOPOROSIS?

No one form of treatment for osteoporosis is universally accepted at this time. Many authorities believe that the combination of calcium supplementation and low-dose estrogen therapy significantly slows or stops bone loss in the immediate postmenopausal period.[12-15] Such treatment should at least prevent a number of vertebral compression fractures.

In most cases this treatment is relatively safe. Problems from treatment with estrogen include an increased incidence of gallbladder disease and the occasional development of endometrial carcinoma, which is an easily detectable and successfully treatable lesion.[12,14] However, many elderly people are concerned about the inconvenience and the expense involved in having to undergo a yearly gynecologic examination to exclude the development of uterine malignancy. A study by Weinstein[12] suggests that estrogen therapy for osteoporosis is cost-effective in patients with prior hysterectomy or documented osteoporosis. It is not cost-effective in asymptomatic individuals without hysterectomy.

Investigators at the Mayo Clinic have successfully utilized treatment with sodium fluoride, calcium, and estrogen. This method has the possible advantage of actually increasing bone mass rather than merely slowing bone loss. Problems with this treatment include fluoride toxicity in some patients and the fact that the added bone is probably of inferior quality.[13]

An approach to treatment we feel deserves further investigation is the development of appropriate exercise programs to strengthen important muscle groups. As mentioned above, decreased muscle strength and defective balance are important contributing factors in femoral fractures. Recently the strength of spinal erector muscles has been shown to be significantly correlated with vertebral bone mineral content.[16] An exercise program may turn out to be an important adjunct to other therapeutic modalities.

Counseling of the patient about creating a safe home environment free of hazards that invite falls is an important part of preventive therapy that should not be omitted.

RECOGNITION ON CONVENTIONAL ROENTGENOGRAMS

Several conventional radiographic findings may be useful in identifying osteoporotic patients in the general population. Barnett and Nordin[17] in 1960 described an osteoporosis index made up of a hand score, a femoral score, and a spine score. The femoral score was equal to 100 times the sum of the medial and lateral femoral cortical thicknesses at the thickest point of the cortex divided by the total width of the shaft at the same point. The hand score was a value similarly derived from measurements at the midpoint of the shaft of the second metacarpal. The spine score was equal to 100 times the ratio of the vertical height of the midportion of the most accurately centered lumbar vertebral body to the anterior height of the same vertebral body. A spine score of 80 or less correlated well with spinal osteoporosis. A hand and femur score of 88 or less correlated well with peripheral osteoporosis. Barnett and Nordin have concluded that their data support the existence of two types of osteoporosis: spinal and peripheral.

Meema[18] in 1963 described a method based on measurement of the combined cortical thickness (CCT) of the radius at its proximal end, just distal to the tuberosity. Using this index, Meema found that women over 76 years of age had a 42-percent reduction in CCT and men a 13-percent reduction. A CCT measurement of less than 5 mm always indicated bone atrophy. Measurements of 2 to 3 mm represented severe osteoporosis. Interestingly, Meema concluded that elderly osteoporotic women with hip fractures did not differ significantly in their degree of osteoporosis from elderly women without fractures.

Anton[19] in 1969 measured the upper cortical thickness of the clavicle at its midpoint. A value of 1.5 mm or less was thought to indicate osteoporosis. The potential usefulness of this measurement is that it can be made on a chest radiograpgh.

End-plate concavity of multiple vertebral bodies, prominent vertebral trabeculation in vertebral bodies, and general loss of density in the midportion of the vertebral bodies are all signs of osteoporosis.[14,20-22] The presence of one or more vertebral compression or other osteoporosis-related fractures also indicates significant osteoporosis. In 1970, Singh[23] proposed changes in the trabecular pattern of the upper end of the femur as an index of osteoporosis. While the Singh index does not correlate well with vertebral fractures, patients with a grade 3 or lower index with discontinuity of the primary tensile trabeculae of the femoral neck almost certainly have severe osteoporosis.

For a more comprehensive account of these qualitative criteria, the reader is referred to recent articles by Wahner and co-workers[24] and Siegelman.[25]

WHY THE CURRENT INTEREST IN OSTEOPOROSIS?

The current high level of interest in the evaluation and treatment of osteoporosis is undoubtedly due to the rising numbers of aged in the population and to the development of newer methods of assessing bone density and/or mineral content as a quantitative index of the condition. Among the most promising of these are photon absorptiometry and quantitative CT. The National Institutes of Health held a consensus development conference on the subject of osteoporosis in 1984, demonstrating the level of national interest in this problem. Articles on the subject are becoming frequent in the lay press. Osteoporosis and osteoporosis-related fractures have been recognized problems for many years. The new instrumentation has given us the hope that it may be possible to recognize individuals prone to osteoporosis-related fractures, prior to the occurrence of such fractures, when treatment of the osteoporosis might be successful in preventing them. The focus of interest in osteoporosis has shifted from the symptomatic patient to the high-risk asymptomatic patient.

A number of devices are now available commercially for the performance of dual photon absorptiometry. Other commercial methods allow conventional CT scanners to perform quantitative bone mineral determinations. The underlying principles of the absorptiometric and CT methods, both of which have been widely publicized as valuable tools for the assessment of the risk of osteoporosis in asymptomatic patients are discussed below. This explanation is followed by a critique of the relative merits and demerits of each of these methods and their relevance to osteoporosis.

ASSESSMENT TECHNIQUES

Single Photon Absorptiometry

The basic principle of this method is shown in Figure 8–1. A narrow beam of monoenergetic photons from a ^{241}Am (60 KeV) or ^{125}I (28 KeV) radioactive source is passed through the organ of interest, usually the distal forearm. The transmitted beam is detected by a NaI crystal coupled to a photomultiplier tube, as the beam traverses linearly across a specified region of the organ. The intensity of the transmitted beam when the beam is intercepted by only the soft tissue component immediately adjacent to bone and the transmitted intensity when the beam is intercepted partly by bone and partly by soft tissue[24] are used to calculate a value for bone mineral. This method has high precision but can only be used for very thin body parts. It is not applicable to measurement of the two most clinically important regions, the femoral neck and spine. This method has been used quite extensively in long-term research projects.

Dual Photon Absorptiometry

The basic principle of this method is the same as that of single photon absorptiometry except that scanning is performed using a ^{153}Gd source that emits two gamma rays during each disintegration (44 and 100 KeV). This permits mathematical compensation for the effect of overlying soft tissues. The method is thus applicable to the femur and spine, the most clinically important regions. Unlike CT, this method does not permit evaluation of trabecular bone independent of cortical bone.

A number of dedicated dual photon absorptiometry (DPA) scanners are commercially available with software and standard normal value data for the lumbar

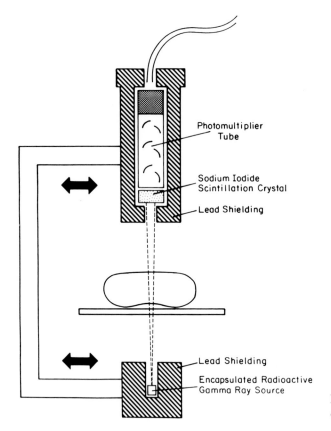

Fig. 8–1. Basic principle of photon absorptiometry.

spine and/or femoral neck. A study requires approximately 15 to 30 minutes. The isotope source must be replaced on a yearly basis.

Single Energy Quantitative CT

The principle of this method as originally developed by Genant et al.[26-29] consists of scanning a patient's lumbar region along with a lucite phantom (Fig. 8–2A) containing varying concentrations of K_2HPO_4 in water placed underneath the patient. K_2HPO_4 is used because it is soluble in water and has an x-ray attenuation coefficient very close to that of the insoluble calcium hydroxyapatite (0.3018 cm²/g versus 0.3124 cm²/g at 70 KeV). Scans are obtained across specific regions of the lumbar spine, usually L2, L3, and L4; the x-ray beam must rotate at right angles to the spinal axis during each scan. This can be easily ensured in modern scanners by first obtaining a pilot or a topographic lateral view and tilting the gantry as needed during the actual scan used for measurements. The patient is made to lie with the hip and the knees flexed to flatten the lumbar spine along the phantom.

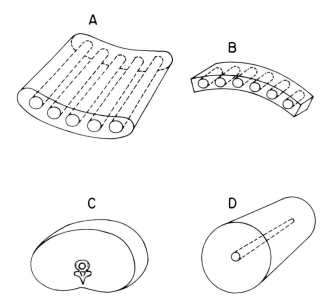

Fig. 8–2. Different types of phantom used in QCT for bone mineral measurement. (A) Phantom used by Genant et al.[26-29] is placed underneath the patient. (B) Phantom used at The Johns Hopkins Hospital is laid on top of the patient. (C) Phantom with a simulated vertebra and a hole in the trabecular region for the insertion of calibration sample is scanned before or after the patient is scanned. (D) A cone-shaped phantom with a hole running through it for the placement of a calibration sample. The conical shape enables one to select a region appropriate for a given patient. A phantom of this type is being developed by the Picker Corporation. It is also scanned before or after a patient.

The CT number obtained with pure water is subtracted from the observed CT numbers to eliminate day-to-day fluctuations in machine calibration. The CT numbers of the K_2HPO_4 samples in the phamtom are used to generate a standard curve of concentration versus CT number. The K_2HPO_4 equivalent of the vertebra can then be read from the standard curve. The Genant phantom

TABLE 8-1. Water content in K_2HPO_4 samples

K_2HPO_4 conc. (mg/cm³)	Water content (mg/cm³)
0	1.000
50	0.992
100	0.973
200	0.951
300	0.919
400	0.889

and software to do the calculations are available commercially. This makes this method quite appealing to those with a CT scanner that is available and not fully utilized for other studies.

Calibration Phantoms

The calibration phantom used in the Genant methods shown in Figure 8–2A is placed beneath the patient on the scanning couch. We have found it a little more convenient to position a curved lucite block (Fig. 8–2B) containing the K_2HPO_4, water, and air samples directly on the patient's abdomen. A number of preliminary tests confirmed that the beam-hardening effects did not introduce any additional error as long as the samples were surrounded by at least 0.25 inches of lucite. It may be argued that, for greater accuracy, a lucite phantom of the same shape and dimensions as the patient should be used, with the calibration samples placed one at a time inside a simulated vertebra within the phantom. Such an approach is being taken by two commercial vendors (Figs. 8–2C, D). While this would be ideal, it would certainly be much more time-consuming, and may not be warranted. Scanning the patient and the phantom separately may introduce additional error, due to interscan variability.

Dual Energy QCT

Here the scanning procedure is the same as for single energy CT except that the scanning is performed at two different kilovoltages. The advantage of this method is the ability to provide accurate bone mineral determinations in patients with large amounts of fat in the marrow space of the bone measured (Fig. 8–3).

The rationale behind this method of calculation is that the soft tissue and fat components within the cancellous region of the bone will yield the same CT number at both the kilovoltages but bone mineral will yield a larger number at the lower kilovoltage. Hence, by taking the difference between the CT number obtained at the two kilovoltages, the problem of the presence of an unknown amount of soft tissue and fat component is eliminated. Unfortunately, as is well known in statistical theory, when two measured numbers are subtracted from each other in a calculation, the uncertainty of the final result increases substantially. On this basis Genant concludes that the accuracy of the method is improved but the precision is reduced by dual energy scanning. Information on implementation of dual energy CT determinations is less readily available than for the single energy method. On many scanners two separate scans of the same slice at different kVp are necessary. This introduces the possibility of motion between scans. Rapid switching of a pulsed beam, described below, offers a solution to this problem but is available on only a few scanners.

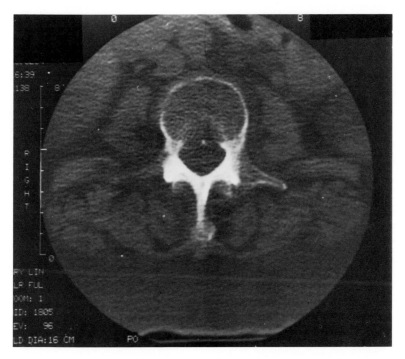

Fig. 8–3. CT scan of a patient with an abnormally high percent of body fat. Note the large fatty deposits even outside the vertebral column. The single energy technique gave negative values for the bone mineral content in this case. (Photo courtesy of Dr. Issa Yaghmai, Medical College of Virginia, Richmond, Virgina.)

Dual Energy CT Methods Based on Basic Physics Principles

The CT methods described thus far are based on scanning a calibration phantom along with the patient or soon thereafter. On the other hand, it is also possible to use the dual energy technique and directly calculate the calcium and the water content in g/cm^3 in each of the pixels included in the scan, provided that the input x-ray spectrum and its attenuation, as it passes through the patient, are explicitly known. In theory, this is possible because the photoelectric and compton cross-sections for calcium and water at various photon energies are accurately known. The details of this methodology are discussed in recent articles by Alvarez, Macovski, and others.[30,31] One problem with this approach is that, in practice, it is not possible to measure the input x-ray spectrum with every patient, so measurements made under laboratory conditions will have to be assumed to be accurate for actual scanning.

In practice it appears to be adequate to ascertain whether the spectrum has deviated by a routine measurement of the half value layer of the beam. Should a significant change be detected, the equipment needs to be recalibrated by a service engineer. Since the calcium and water content are determined on a per pixel basis it is essential that any patient motion or relative gantry motion between scans be eliminated. Practically speaking, this means that both scans be done within the same "breath-holding" by the patient. Also, due to normal mechanical stresses, scans done with rotation in opposite directions often do not superimpose perfectly. One manufacturer (Siemens), which produces third generation systems with a pulsed x-ray beam, has implemented a unique solution. This design pulses the x-ray beam alternately at high and low kVp values, thus obtaining two projection data sets in a single scan. This method shows considerable promise although it is probably restricted to third-generation pulsed x-ray systems. Furthermore, this method enables the computation of bone mineral in terms of elemental calcium and not in terms of calcium hydroxyapatite or its radiographic equivalent, K_2HPO_4. Apart from this, the procedure may also be expected to result in significant errors due to the fact that the computations are made under the assumption that the region of interest contains only calcium and water whereas, in practice, there is bound to be an unknown mixture of fat, soft tissue, and bone mineral. The method's intrinsic advantages, however, are that calibration samples need not be scanned with the patient and the method is relatively immune to beam hardening artifacts that impart a positional dependence on the obtained CT numbers.

Comparison of the Absorptiometric and the CT Methods

As already noted, the single photon absorptiometric method (SPA) yields the total (cancellous and trabecular) bone mass in units of gm/cm of the length of the bone scanned. This implies that great care has to be exercised, in practice, to ensure that identical regions of the organ are scanned in all patients. Furthermore, accurate repositioning of the body part is extremely important, especially if longitudinal studies on the same patient are intended. For these reasons, SPA is usually limited to appendicular sites such as the radius. Several technical innovations such as multiple scans, use of laser beams for repositioning accuracy, and use of a water bath to maintain a constant soft tissue thickness have improved the accuracy of this measurement in recent years. Most manufacturers claim an accuracy of ± 5 percent with their instruments. The spine and femur, which are of most current practical interest, cannot be examined.

The dual photon absorptiometric method (DPA) yields total (cancellous and trabecular) bone mass (g) along the path of the photon beam per cm^2 at right angles to the beam. The values obtained depend considerably, as with SPA, on patient positioning In addition, significant errors are introduced if the photon beam happens to be intercepted by metallic objects, soft tissue calcifications such as the calcified aortic wall, or contrast-enhancing agents such as barium in the gastrointestinal tract. While DPA is usually employed for evaluating the average bone mass (BMC) in g/cm^2 in the region of L1 to L4 vertebrae, it has also been employed in the evaluation of the proximal femur. Also, since this method does not give a clear image of the spine such as is obtained with the CT topogram, the conscientious practitioner would probably want to obtain a plain radiographic view of the spine as well to avoid overlooking fractures, metastatic lesions, and other important incidental findings that could be confused with osteoporosis.

Quantitative computed tomography (QCT) can, in principle, be used to measure either cancellous bone or cortical bone. In practice, however, it is most commonly used to evalutate the bone mineral content of cancellous bone in L1 to L4 vertebrae. In the case of Genant's method of calibration, the result is given directly in g/cm^3 of K_2HPO_4 equivalent which, as stated before, has radiographic attenuation characteristics almost identical to those of calcium hydroxyapatite. In the case of the Alvarez and Macovski method, the result is given in g/cm^3 of elemental calcium. The two methods differ, the calcium content being lower by a constant factor. Rohloff et al.[32] have estimated this factor to be 1.8 for the calcaneus and 2.5 for vertebral cancellous bone.

Quantitative CT is not as sensitive to positioning difficulties as SPA and DPA and can be easily performed on any good CT scanner. While it does not require the purchase of any additional equipment, it does require the availability of an appropriate phantom and software to perform the calculations. It can be used to evaluate either the appendicular skeleton or the axial skeleton or both and the result is always in g/cm^3 K_2HPO_4, which is conceptually a better index than the g/cm of SPA or the g/cm^2 of DPA. The ability of CT to evaluate the metabolically active trabecular bone independently is thought by many to be advantageous. However, CT scans are, to date, more expensive than SPA and DPA measurements ($300 versus $150). Also the radiation dose is much larger with today's scanners (1 to 3 rads versus 20 to 30 mrad). A practitioner should be able to estimate the scanner time required to perform a study; it should be shorter than for DPA.

Single energy CT provides greater precision than dual energy CT and can be performed on nearly all scanners. It is subject to large errors in patients with a high fat content in the marrow.

Dual energy CT provides better accuracy at the expense of lower precision. Only certain scanners can perform successful dual energy studies.

DISCUSSION AND CONCLUSIONS

The technology of bone mineral and/or density measurements, as discussed in this chapter, has advanced to the point that measurement reproducibilities with ±2 percent can be obtained with a comparable level of accuracy if repeated measurements are made of a standard sample placed within a phantom. Several ways of improving the accuracy even further are on the horizon.[33] The same degree of accuracy, however, is often difficult to achieve in actual patient measurements. In practice, the accuracy drops to about 20 percent. Obviously this degree of accuracy is not adequate, since it is known that the rate of bone loss is only of the order of about 1 percent per year. Furthermore, as noted before, measurements made with the different techniques are dimensionally different. Intrainstrumental differences that have not been fully explored may also exist.

A number of investigators have attempted to obtain normal values of the bone mineral content measured by different methods as a funciton of age and sex (Fig. 8–4). These studies have shown that within the same age bracket, the standard deviation of the mean can be as much as ± 20 percent and that considerable overlap exists between normal and clearly osteoporotic patients. For this reason, the concept of a threshold value below which a patient is to be considered osteoporotic has been proposed.[34,35] In the case of DPA, Riggs et al.[34] recommend a threshold value of 965 mg/cm² and in the case of QCT,

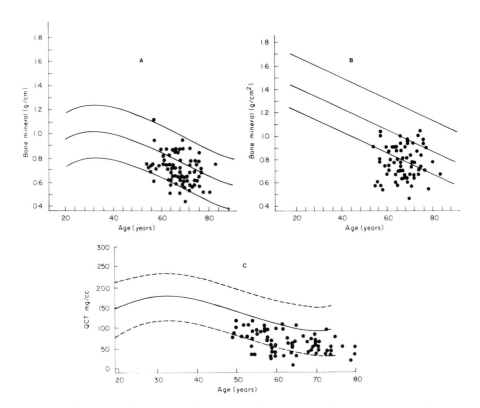

Fig. 8–4. Measured bone mineral content of women with osteoporosis and one or more vertebral—compression fractures (dots). (A) Measurement of the distal radius (SPA method). (B) Measurement of the lumbar spine (DPA method). (C) Measurement of the lumbar spine (QCT method). The center curve in each diagram gives the mean values for normal women as a function of age. The upper and the lower curves represent the 90 percent confidence limits. Note the considerable overlap of the osteoporotics with normals. (Data from Riggs BL, Wahner HW, Dunn WL et al: Differential changes in bone mineral density of the appendicular and axial skeleton with aging. J Clin Invest 67:328, 1981; Genant HK: Osteoporosis: advanced radiologic assessment using quantitative computed tomography. Western J Med July: 84, 1983.)

Genant[35] recommends a value of 105 mg/cm^3 for compression fractures of the spine. While this may be of some value, it must be recognized that breaking strength and fracture risk are complex functions not only of the mineral content of cortical and trabecular bone but also of geometric and architectural irregularities. Still another complication in SPA done on an extremity is that changes in the appendicular skeleton are not necessarily reflected in the axial skeleton.[27]

A further point is that after age 30 or so, there is a steady yearly decline of 1 to 3 percent not only of bone mineral but also of many other physiologic parameters such as cardiac function, glomerular filtration rate, and breathing capacity. Susceptibility to infections and the incidence of cancer, heart disease, and autoimmune diseases such as rheumatoid arthritis are also known to rise dramatically with age. Thus it appears that there is a general decline of homeostatic control with age. Attempts to correct particular deficiencies should be viewed in this light.

On top of all these considerations there is already a tremendous concern over the escalation of health care costs. Bone mineral measurements are expensive and often are not conclusive. With the present state of the art and clinical knowledge, screening everyone for osteoporosis is certainly not indicated. It may, however, be possible from other routine clinical investigations to select groups of high-risk patients. It is also possible, using conventional radiographic examinations, to detect patients with probable osteoporosis who might need a more accurate bone density determination. At the same time it does not seem unreasonable to institute treatment of some high-risk patients on the basis of clinical findings alone without any bone density determinations. However, as discussed earlier, current therapies for management of potential osteoporosis have their own uncertainties and complications.

In view of these various uncertainties, we believe that the measurement of bone mineral content and the institution of therapy based on such measurement are still in the investigational stage and any attempt to institute mass screening programs should wait until more accurate evaluations and definitive therapies become available. For additional views on this controversial subject, the reader is referred to recent articles by Cann[36] and Avioli,[37] and the review by the Health and Public Policy Committee of the American College of Physicians.[38]

REFERENCES

1. Richelson LS, Wahner HW, Melton LJ et al: Relative contributions of aging and estrogen deficiency to postmenopausal bone loss. N Engl J Med 311:1273, 1984
2. Cann CE, Genant HK, Ettinger B et al: Spinal mineral loss in oophorectomized women. JAMA 244:2056, 1980
3. Trotter M, Broman GE, Peterson RR: Densities of bones of white and negro skeletons. J Bone Joint Surg 42A:50, 1960
4. Johnston CC, Jr: Identification of population susceptible to osteoporosis. Abstract: National Institutes of Health Consensus Development Conference, April 2–4, 1984, pp. 29–31
5. Rigotti NA, Nussbaum SR, Herzog DB et al: Osteoporosis in women with anorexia nervosa. N Engl J Med 311:1601, 1984

6. Cann EC, Martin MC, Genant HK et al: Decreased spinal mineral content in amenorrheic women. JAMA 251:626, 1984

7. Iskrant AP, Smith RW, Jr: Osteoporosis in women 45 years and over related to subsequent fractures. Public Health Rep 84:33, 1969

8. Urist MR: Orthopaedic management of osteoporosis in postmenopausal women. Clin Endocrinol Metab 2:159, 1973

9. Boucher CA: Accidents among old persons. Geriatrics 14:293, 1959

10. Overstall PW, Exton-Smith AN, Imms FJ et al: Falls in the elderly related to postural imbalance. Br Med J 1:261, 1977

11. Pogrund H, Makin M, Robin G et al: Osteoporosis in patients with fractured femoral neck in Jerusalem. Clin Orthop Rel Res 124:165, 1977

12. Weinstein MC: Estrogen use in postmenopausal women—costs, risks, and benefits. N Engl J Med 303:308, 1980

13. Riggs BL, Seeman E, Hodgson SF et al: Effect of the fluoride/calcium regimen on vertebral fracture occurrence in postmenopausal osteoporosis. N Engl J Med 306:446, 1982

14. Henneman PH, Wallach S: The use of androgens and estrogens and their metabolic effects: a review of the prolonged use of estrogens and androgens in postmenopausal and senile osteoporosis. Arch Intern Med 100:715, 1957

15. Ettinger B, Genant HK, Cann C: Menopause bone loss can be prevented by low dose estrogen with calcium supplements. J Comput Assist Tomogr 9:633, 1985

16. Sinaki M, McPhee MC, Hodgson SF et al: Relationship between bone mineral density of spine and strength of buck extensors in healthy postmenopausal women. Mayo Clin Proc 61:116, 1986

17. Barnett E, Nordin BEC: The radiological diagnosis of osteoporosis: a new approach. Clin Radiol 11:166, 1960

18. Meema HE: Cortical bone atrophy and osteoporosis as a manifestation of aging. Am J Roentgenol 89: 1287, 1963

19. Anton HC: Width of clavicular cortex in osteoporosis. Br Med J 1:409, 1969

20. Caldwell RA, Collins DH: Assessment of vertebral osteoporosis by radiographic and chemical methods post-mortem. J Bone Joint Surg 43B: 34, 1961

21. Saville PD: A quantitative approach to simple radiographic diagnosis of osteoporosis: its application to the osteoporosis of rheumatoid arthritis. Arthritis Rheum 10:416, 1967

22. Boukhris R, Becker KL: The inter-relationship between vertebral fractures and osteoporosis. Clin Orthop Rel Res 90:209, 1973

23. Singh M, Nagrath AR, Maini PS: Changes in trabecular pattern of the upper end of the femur as an index of osteoporosis. J Bone Joint Surg 52A:457, 1970

24. Wahner HW, Dunn W, Riggs BL: Non-invasive bone mineral measurements. Semin Nucl Med 13:282, 1983

25. Siegelman, SS: The radiology of osteoporosis. p. 68. In Brazil US (ed): Osteoporosis. Grune and Stratton, New York, 1970

26. Cann CE, Genant HK: Precise measurement of vertebral mineral content using computed tomography. J Comput Assist Tomogr 4:493, 1980

27. Genant HK, Boyd DP: Quantitative bone mineral analysis using dual-energy computed tomography. Invest Radiol 12:545, 1977

28. Cann CE, Genant HK, Young DR: Comparison of vertebral and peripheral mineral losses in disuse osteoporosis in monkeys. Radiology 134:525, 1980

29. Genant HK, Cann CE, Ettinger B et al: Quantitative computed tomography of vertebral spongiosa: a sensitive method for detecting early bone loss after oophorectomy. Ann Intern Med 97:699, 1982

30. Alvarez RE, Macovski A: Energy selective reconstructions in x-ray computerized tomography. Phys Med Biol 21:733–744, 1971

31. Isherwood I, Pullau BR, Rutherford RA, Straug FA: Electron density and atomic number determination by computed tomography. Br J Radiol 50:613, 1977

32. Rohloff R, Arndt W, Hitzler H, Frey KW: Experimental studies on accuracy and precision of CT mineral determination in human trabecular cadaver bones. J Comput Assist Tomogr 9:604, 1985

33. Rutt BK, Stebler BG, Cann CE et al: Whole-body CT scanner for ultra-precise, ultra-accurate determination of bone density. J Comput Assist Tomogr 9:609, 1985

34. Riggs BL, Wahner HW, Dunn WL et al: Differential changes in bone mineral density of the appendicular and axial skeleton with aging. J Clin Invest 67:328, 1981

35. Genant HK: Osteoporosis: advanced radiologic assessment using quantitative computed tomography. Western J Med July: 84, 1983

36. Cann CE. Commentary: Do we need sophisticated measurements for bone mineral analysis. J Comput Assist Tomogr 9:639, 1985

37. Avioli LV. Osteoporosis: let's look at the facts. Geriatrics 39:16, 1984

38. Health and Public Policy Committee, American College of Physicians: Radiologic methods to evaluate bone mineral content. Ann Intern Med 100:908, 1984

9 MRI of The Musculoskeletal System

STEVEN E. HARMS

The early applications of magnetic resonance imaging (MRI) were primarily aimed at the diagnosis of neurologic problems. Initial studies ignored the musculoskeletal system primarily because of the inability of MRI to resolve bone directly.[1-8] More recently the high-quality soft tissue anatomical and physiologic information provided by MRI has been recognized as a significant adjunct to the conventional diagnostic work-up of many musculoskeletal disorders.[9-13]

In this chapter the basic principles of MRI and technique selection are outlined. These principles are applied to the solution of clinical problems encountered in the diagnosis of musculoskeletal diseases.

PRINCIPLES

The basic physics of MRI have been reviewed in detail by many authors.[14-26] The principles needed to understand musculoskeletal applications are outlined here.

Some nuclear species, when placed in the appropriate radiofrequency and magnetic fields, can resonantly absorb energy and produce a radiofrequency signal; hence the name *magnetic resonance* (MR). Because of its high abundance within most body tissues and high MR signal, hydrogen is the nucleus used by most clinical imagers.

Signals obtained from hydrogen nuclei (protons) in MRI are dependent upon a variety of parameters.[27] The proton density ($N(H)$) refers to the relative number of resonating nuclei per given region. Either macroscopic flow[28-32] or microscopic diffusion[33,34] also affects the MR signal intensity. The chemical shift results in a shift in resonance frequency due to the chemical environment of the resonating nucleus. In proton imaging, the chemical shift is best known for the shift in fat signals relative to water signals, resulting in an artifact in the frequency-encoded direction. This phenomenon has also been used to obtain separate fat and water images.[35-37]

The most important determinants of tissue contrast in proton magnetic resonance imaging are the relaxation times, T_1 and T_2 (Fig. 9-1). Spin-lattice relaxation, characterized by the time constant T_1, results from the dissipation of energy by excited nuclei through thermal interactions with the environment. Spin-spin relaxation, characterized by the time constant T_2, is a result of energy exchange between nuclei.[38-43]

The chemical environment of the nuclei affects their relaxation behavior. A number of theories have been proposed to explain the differences in relaxation times of tissue.[44-47] A simplified explanation of the possible mechanism is provided. Most of the signal from protons within the tissue comes from the hydrogen nuclei of water molecules. Suppose water existed in two phases, a "free" phase and a "bound" phase. In the "free" phase, the water molecules are freely tumbling, and energy exchange to adjacent molecules is hindered. In this environment, slower relaxation would be expected. In the "bound" state, water molecules are closely associated with the charges on adjacent proteins and their molecular motion is impaired. Because of the relationship to the adjacent macromolecules, the "bound" water more readily dissipates energy to the adjacent macromolecules, resulting in faster relaxation. Cells are composed of a combination of soluble components, low-molecular-weight solutes, and immobilized macromolecular assemblies. The relative distribution of water in these phases will reflect the overall relaxation times of the tissue.

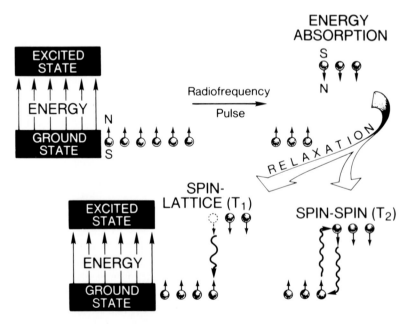

FIG. 9-1. T_1 and T_2. Spin-lattice relaxation, characterized by the time constant T_1, is the result of thermal interactions of excited nuclei with the environment. In spin-spin relaxation, energy is exchanged between nuclei. Spin-spin relaxation is described by the time constant, T_2. (Harms SE, Morgan TJ, Yamanashi WS et al: Principles of nuclear magnetic resonance imaging. RadioGraphics 4:26, 1984.)

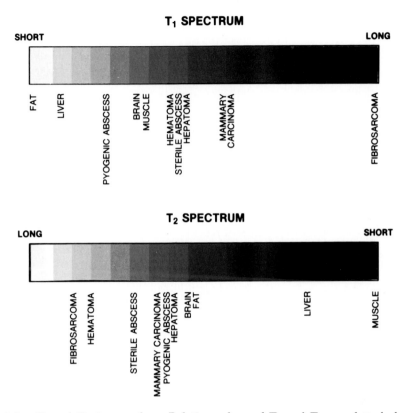

FIG. 9-2. T_1 and T_2 tissue values. Relative values of T_1 and T_2 are plotted along a spectrum. Short T_1 and long T_2 usually result in high signal on their respective weighted images while long T_1 and short T_2 usually result in low signal. (Reprinted with permission from Harms SE, Kramer DM: Fundamentals of magnetic resonance. CRC Crit Rev Diagn Imaging 25:79, 1985. Copyright, CRC Press, Inc., Boca Raton, FL)

In 1971, Damadian[48] observed that the T_1 of some tumor tissues was significantly longer than the corresponding normal tissues. While the explanation for this finding remains controversial, the general tendency toward longer T_1 values in tumors is well accepted[49-52] and was the incentive behind the development of MRI.[53] When the relaxation times of a larger number of tissues are compared, a broad spectrum of relaxation behavior is found among tissues.[54] Although a number of tumors without significant prolongation of the relaxation times compared to normal tissue have been found, the tremendous contrast afforded by MR can still be used to great advantage by producing superb soft tissue image detail. The relative values of T_1 and T_2 for a variety of pathologic and normal tissues are plotted on a spectrum in Figure 9-2. By most imaging methods, a short T_1 and long T_2 tissue has higher signal intensity than a long T_1 and short T_2 tissue. Therefore, compared to the T_1 spectrum, the T_2 spectrum is reversed with short T_1 and long T_2 toward the high-intensity

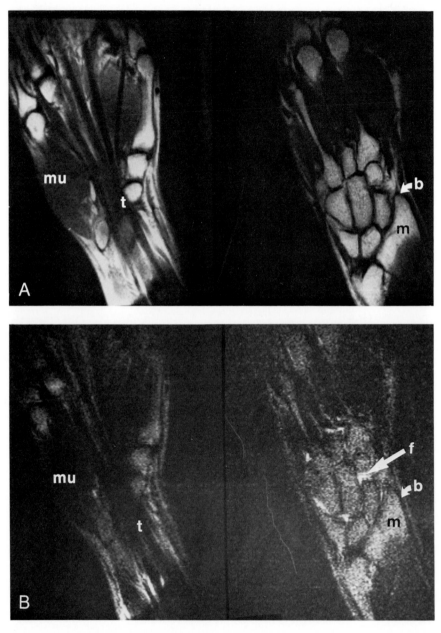

FIG. 9-3. Normal wrist images. The marrow fat (m), muscle (mu), cortical bone (b), tendon (t), and joint fluid (f) are labeled on (A) T_1-, (B) T_2-, and (C) N(H)-weighted images of a normal wrist. The highly T_2 weighted images have low signal but many lesions are enhanced because of their long T_2.

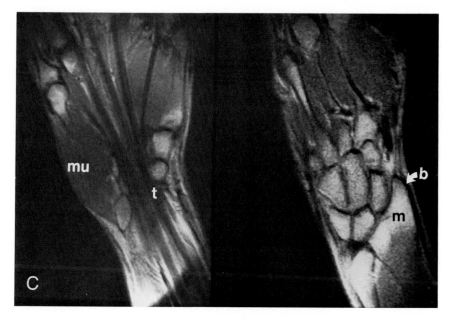

FIG. 9-3. (*continued*).

end of the scale and long T_1 and short T_2 toward the low-intensity end of the scale.

Most tumors have a long T_1 and T_2. In terms of intensity, these tumors would be on the low signal side of the T_1 spectrum but on the high signal side of the T_2 spectrum. Muscle has an intermediate T_1 but a very short T_2 (low signal). Fat has a short T_1 (high signal) and a moderate T_2.[55]

A set of wrist images from a normal volunteer shows the usual appearance of tissue signals on T_1-, T_2-, and N(H)-weighted images (Fig. 9-3). Fat has high signal on the T_1-weighted images, moderately low signal on the T_2-weighted images, and moderately high signal on the N(H)-weighted images. Muscle has moderate signal on the T_1- and N(H)-weighted images but very low signal on the T_2-weighted images. Cortical bone has low signal on all images because of a short T_2 and low N(H). Tendons have low signal on all images because of a very short T_2. Joint fluid is highlighted on the T_2-weighted images because of the prolonged T_2 of the fluid. Despite the more noisy appearance, the T_2 images can also be used to define tumor masses better because of their long T_2.

TECHNIQUE

Magnetic resonance imaging is a very flexible modality with an almost limitless number of technique choices. The MRI specialist should have a technique plan in mind to fit the clinical setting and some contingency plans available

TABLE 9-1. Major technique categories of MRI

Radiofrequency coil
Head
Body
Breast
Surface
Other
Pulse sequence
Single spin echo
Multiple spin echo
Inversion spin echo
Timing parameter
TE
TR
TI
Acquisition methods
2DFT single slice
2DFT multislice
Nonselective 3DFT
Isotropic
Anisotropic
Selective 3DFT
Isotropic
Anisotropic
Selective 3DFT multislab
2D and 3D hybrid echo-planar

if the situation changes during the imaging process. Some of the considerations needed to make the decisions are outlined here.

Technical parameters requiring selection include radiofrequency (rf) coil, pulse sequence, timing parameters, and acquisition method (Table 9-1). These categories are all interrelated. Making a change in one choice may require changes in other areas. The attributes of the various techniques are compared and contrasted below.

Radiofrequency Coil

Initial MR imagers were provided with a head coil for head and extremity imaging and a body coil for the rest of the body. A variety of other coils for specialized purposes have recently been developed.[56-58] Most of these coils are called surface coils because of their placement in proximity to the skin surface.[59-62] Their basic advantage is localization of signal from a small desired region with the reduction of unwanted signals and noise from the rest of the body. These coils thus improve the signal to noise ratio (S/N) for images of smaller regions.

A coil that covers only the desired region of interest is generally considered ideal. A wrist would, therefore, be better imaged by a smaller coil than a knee. The pelvis would require either a very large surface coil or the body coil.

The transmit and receiver functions of the coil may be performed by the same coil or separately. A small receiver surface coil combined with transmission by the body coil is the most favored configuration. Transmission by the body coil results in a usually more homogeneous radiofrequency field. Larger transmit coils, however, could result in greater rf power deposition, which may limit the number of slices or echoes according to current recommended power limits.[63] This problem is more severe at higher field strengths. Since the larger transmit coils require more power, nonselective three-dimensional acquisitions are limited by the transmitter power supply.

Using the same coil to transmit and receive usually results in a more inhomogeneous transmitted field. This situation could be advantageous in saturating unwanted signals near the coil. These coils usually have a different design to compensate for the combined transmit and receive functions. Transmit and receive solonoid surface coils have been effectively used to image extremities in permanent magnet systems.[62] Solonoid coils have a more homogeneous transmitted field than typical surface coils. Unfortunately, these coils would be difficult to use in superconducting magnets since the magnetic flux in these magnets is oriented down the axis of the magnet tube and the rf field needs to be orthogonal to the static magnetic field.

Pulse Sequences and Timing Parameters

These two technique choices are discussed together since they are closely related.

A number of pulse sequences are possible, but currently only three are available on most production machines: single spin-echo, multiple spin-echo, and inversion spin-echo.[15,21-26] Echo time (TE) and repetition time (TR) are used to describe the single spin-echo (Fig. 9-4) and multiple spin-echo sequences (Fig. 9-5). For the inversion spin-echo sequence, the inversion time (TI) is added. The TI is the time interval between the 180° inversion pulse and the 90° pulse of the spin echo sequence.

The signal intensity, I, for a given echo, k, obtained at TE_k is described by the equation:

$$I = N(H) \ f(v) \ [1-\exp-(TR-TE_n)/T_1](\exp-TE_k/T_2) \tag{1}$$

where $N(H)$ is the proton density, $f(v)$ is the flow-related function, and TE_n is the TE of the last echo of a multiecho sequence. As the TE_k increases, the

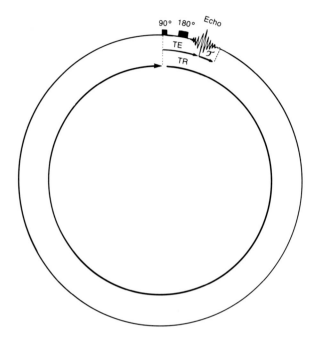

FIG. 9-4. Single spin echo sequence. The echo time (TE) defines the time between the 90° pulse and the middle of the echo. The repetition time TR is the time from the beginning of the 90° pulse to the beginning of the 90° pulse of the next sequence. The echo signal lasts a period of time (τ) past the midpoint. (Harms SE, Siemers PT, Hildenbrand P, Plum G: Multiple spin echo magnetic resonance imaging of the brain. RadioGraphics 6(1):117, 1986.)

signal intensity decreases due to T_2-weighting. Only the TE_k affects the T_2-related component of the equation. The T_1 weighting is increased by decreasing the $TR-TE_n$ term. This decrease can be achieved by either shortening the TR or lengthening the echo train (TE_n). If both a short TR and a long echo train are used, then the entire sequence will be T_1-weighted (low $TR-TE_n$) and the

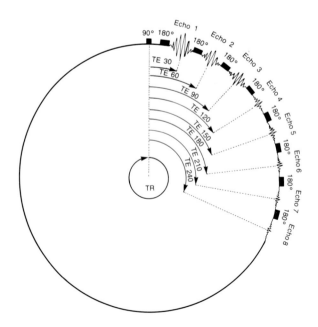

FIG. 9-5. Multiple spin echo sequence. A series of eight 180° pulses are applied in this example to obtain a set of signals at different TEs within the same sequence. A larger portion of the TR cycle is used to obtain addition echoes. (Harms SE, Siemers PT, Hildenbrand P, Plum G: Multiple spin echo magnetic resonance imaging of the brain. RadioGraphics, 6(1):117, 1986.)

longer TE echoes of the echo train will become progressively T_2-weighted. Therefore, both T_1- and T_2-weighted images can be achieved in the same multi-echo sequence at the expense of an overall reduced signal.[64,65] If the TE_n is short and the TR is long, then reduced T_1 and T_2 weighting is achieved. A sufficiently short TE_k and long TR results in a predominance of the N(H) component of the equation for proton density weighted images. A multiecho sequence with a sufficiently long TR results in a N(H)-weighted first echo with increased T_2 weighting for each additional echo.

The inversion spin echo sequence is typically used to enhance T_1 weighting of a spin echo sequence through the use of an inversion pulse prior to the spin echo. The signal intensity for the kth echo of an inversion spin echo sequence is described by the equation:

$$I = N(H)f(v)[1-(2-exp-(TR-TI-TE_n)/T_1)exp-TI/T_1]exp-TE_k/T_2 \qquad (2)$$

where TI is the inversion time and the other parameters are defined as in the equation (1). T_1 weighting is typically achieved by shortening the TI so as to decrease the TI/T_1 portion of the equation. T_1 weighting can also be enhanced by decreasing the $TR-TI-TE_n$ term either through a shorter TR or a longer TI and TE_n. T_2 weighting is the same as in the spin echo sequence where an increased TE_k results in more T_2 dependence.

Acquisition Methods

Fourier transform (FT) imaging in either the two-dimensional (2D) mode or the three-dimensional (3D) mode is the basis of most commercial image acquisitions. With this method, phase-encoding and frequency-encoding gradients are used to localize MR signals and produce an MR image. Two-dimensional methods use single phase- and frequency-encoding gradients. The 3D methods use two phase-encoding gradients and a single frequency-encoding gradient. The acquisition methods commonly used commercially include 2DFT single slice, 2DFT multislice, nonselective 3DFT, and selective 3DFT. These methods and their relationship to the other technique choices are discussed below and several emerging methods are also described.

2DFT

Almost all MR imagers use the 2DFT method. A 2D slice is selected with an excitation pulse in the presence of a magnetic field gradient.[66] The scan time, t, for a 2DFT acquisition is described by the equation:

$$t = (nN) \, TR \qquad (3)$$

where N is the number of phase-encoded projections and n is the number of excitations. The scan time is approximately the same for all manufacturers.

To improve efficiency, the 2D multislice method was developed.[67] Since the time required to acquire the echo is usually short compared to the TR of the pulse sequence, additional 2D slices can be excited sequentially throughout the remaining TR interval while the first slice recovers. The maximum number of slices, S_{max}, per scan is described by the equation:

$$S_{max} = TR/E_a \qquad (4)$$

where the E_a is the time required to acquire the echo signal. The E_a is the sum of the TE_n, the time from the middle of the echo to the end of the echo (approximately $\frac{1}{2}$ TE of the shortest echo), and a dead time determined largely by gradient cooling. The dead time varies with the manufacturer. The S_{max} decreases with a shorter TR and/or a longer E_a. A longer E_a results from a longer TE_n or a longer dead time.

The 2D multislice acquisition method is most efficient for long TR, short TE pulse sequences where more slices are available. It is an effective method therefore for N(H)- and moderately T_2-weighted pulse sequences. When one is using a multiecho sequence, a longer TR is often required to obtain a reasonable number of slices with a long TE_n. The images from this sequence will vary from an N(H)-weighted image with short TE to increasingly T_2-weighted images with longer TE.

T_1 weighting is more difficult to achieve with 2D multislice. When one is using a spin echo sequence, T_1 weighting requires a short $TR-TE_n$ and a short TE_k. An adequate number of slices for a given region of interest may be difficult especially if the instrument has a long dead time. For example, a TE 30, TR 500 pulse sequence with a E_a of 100 msec would yield only five slices. If the E_a could be reduced to 50 msec then 10 slices could be performed. For T_1-weighting purposes, a TE 15, TR 300 would be better, but an E_a of 50 msec would yield only six slices. If the TE was reduced to 15 msec and the dead time reduced for an E_a of 30, then 10 slices could be obtained in the same TR 300 sequence. The importance of a short TE and reduced dead time, in terms of acquisition efficiency, is apparent.

Due to the shape of the slice selection pulses and signal saturation by adjacent slices, gaps are placed between slices. The acquisition of thin slices is often limited by the gradient strength. The slices can be made thinner at the expense of a longer TE. Very thin slices may require a larger slice gap. Paradoxic enhancement in vessels is frequently seen in 2D multislice acquisitions. Paradoxically high signal is seen in vessels due to the incoming flow of less saturated blood into a slice with relatively saturated tissue.[68]

3DFT

True 3D acquisitions are possible on some commercial instruments. In 3DFT, slices are resolved using an additional phase-encoding gradient. The voxel can be equal on all three sides (isotropic) or resolution can be sacrificed in the slice-encoding direction (anisotropic). The 3DFT methods can be further divided into nonselective and selective modes. The nonselective 3D acquisition refers to the application of the excitation to the entire volume of the rf coil in the absence of a magnetic field gradient. The selective 3D acquisition refers to the use of a selective rf excitation of a volume of tissue in the presence of a gradient. The selective 3D method limits the acquisition to a smaller volume within the rf coil.[15]

The scan time, s, for a 3D acquisition can be approximated by the equation

$$s = (nNS)TR \tag{5}$$

where S is the number of slices per scan and N is the number of in slice phase-encoding projections. Since the signal to noise ratio (S/N) increases with the square root of S, there is usually no need for additional excitations and n is usually 1. If unipolar phase-encoding is used, a phase reconstruction can be used to reduce N and the scan time by about half for the same resolution. Since the scan time increases with TR, 3D acquisitions favor short TR sequences. The number of slices per scan is not reduced by a shorter TR or longer TE as in 2D multislice. Since slices are obtained by phase encoding instead of selective excitation, there is no slice gap. Phase encoding also allows the production of very thin slices with lower gradient strengths. Very uniform tip angles are present in the center slices for better S/N. The S/N can also be improved with the use of nonselective 180° rf pulses. Paradoxic enhancement is reduced especially when large volumes of tissue are excited.

Miscellaneous Methods

Projection reconstruction (PR) was used to produce the first MR images[53] and is the standard method for acquiring CT images. Due to certain limitations of scan time and artifact formation, PR is not widely used for MR proton imaging at present. Because of the ability of PR to image free induction decay (FID) signals, this method could again be used for the imaging of very short T_2 spins such as ^{19}F or ^{23}Na where a spin echo sequence would result in a substantial signal loss due to T_2.

The use of a selective 3D acquisition in a "multislab" mode has been proposed.[69] This method uses the TR interval for the selective excitation of multiple 3D "slabs" similar to a 2D multislice. The selected slabs are further divided into slices by phase-encoding gradients in a typical 3DFT manner. The efficiency of multislice would be combined with the high S/N, thin slice, short TR, and long TE capability of 3D.

Rapid switching of the gradients can achieve very fast echoes. If the T_2 is long compared to the echo time, then several echoes can be acquired from the same excitation. Based on this principle, the number of phase-encoding projections can be reduced or eliminated to achieve a faster scan time. If no phase-encoding is used, this method is called echo planar imaging.[70] When this method is combined with the phase-encoding of FT imaging, it is called hybrid echo planar imaging.[71] The echo planar method is designed to speed image acquisitions. Scan times of 64 mseconds per frame produced cine images of the beating heart using this method.[72]

CLINICAL APPLICATIONS

The application of MRI in the diagnosis of musculoskeletal disorders utilizes the entire range of technique choices. The detailed imaging required for visualization of small carpal bone abnormalities is quite different from the technique used for a metastatic spine survey. T_1 and T_2 information may provide the specificity needed for the diagnosis of a soft tissue mass, but would not be useful in quantifing the size of an anterior cruciate tear. The region of the body and the clinical setting will dictate the design of the MR exam. The flexibility of MR makes the tailoring of the procedure a diagnostic necessity. In this rapidly emerging field, new information is gained almost daily. A framework for the thought process needed in designing the MR examination is provided. As knowledge of MR applications increase, additional data can be integrated into the overall imaging scheme.

Bone and Soft Tissue Tumors

Anatomy

A method for imaging high-resolution tomographic anatomy with high soft tissue contrast is needed for the accurate staging of bone and soft tissue neoplasms. Magnetic resonance does not provide the bony detail offered by radiographic methods, but the soft tissue anatomy is usually far superior.[9-13,73-76] In addition, the ability of MR to acquire images directly from multiple imaging planes is a significant advantage in evaluating extremities.

The signal intensity patterns of the normal musculoskeletal tissues are well differentiated. As described earlier, most tumor tissues have signal patterns that are quite different from surrounding tissues. In order for one to stage the lesion accurately, the bone marrow, vessels, nerves, joints, and bony cortex need to be well visualized.

The high-signal bone marrow provides excellent contrast on T_1-weighted images. Most tumors have a longer T_1 and lower signal than fat on T_1-weighted images. An example of this contrast is shown with a metastatic melanoma of the spine (Fig. 9-6). Very T_2 weighted images have diminished signal from fat compared to many tumors and edema, as discussed earlier. The metastatic lesions have lower signal than fat on the T_1-weighted images but higher signal than fat on the high T_2-weighted images. In the case shown, the radiographs and bone scan were negative. Lesions missed by bone scan and radiographs have also been seen in metastatic breast and lung carcinoma. Early results indicate that MRI may be the most sensitive imaging modality in the evaluation of bone marrow disease.[72,75,76]

Vessels and nerves are often difficult to define on CT. The vessels can be seen by angiography, but the definition of the mass extent is more difficult. Flowing blood within vessels usually contributes little signal in MR images except in cases of paradoxic enhancement. Paradoxic enhancement results in

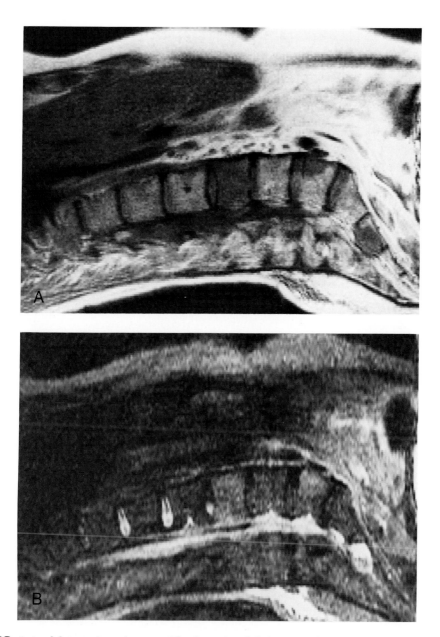

FIG. 9-6.   Metastatic melanoma. The low signal defects on the (A) T_1-weighted (TE 30, TR 500) image and high signal areas on the (B) T_2-weighted (TE 120, TR 2000) within the vertebral bodies demonstrate metastatic melanoma that was not identified on either the CT or the radionuclide bone scan. The 2DFT multislice acquisition was obtained using the body coil.

higher signal from the vessel due to fresh unsaturated blood flowing into the slice.[77] This phenomenon is typically seen in 2D multislice techniques toward the ends of the acquisition. MR can provide good anatomic definition of both vascular anatomy and the lesion at the same time (Fig. 9-7). This information is very helpful in surgical cases where a limb salvage procedure could be performed.

The high soft tissue contrast and direct sagittal imaging aids in the definition of muscle bundles and fascial planes. Soft tissue neoplasms such as the malignant fibrous histiocytoma shown in Figure 9-8 tend to extend up and down fascial planes. Edema has high signal on T2-weighted images. This information is very helpful in the accurate staging of these lesions since tumor cells often spread with the edema. Definition of a mass lesion is usually necessary for CT staging, but the signal intensity variations noted on MR will more correctly define the extent of the tumor and edema within the fascial planes, even in the absence of a defined mass.

Tissue Characteristics

At the present state of technology, the ability of MR images to characterize tissue is primitive.[11-13] T_1-, T_2-, and N(H)-weighted images can be obtained by the methods described previously. Because of the wide variation of pathologic tissue change that occurs in this region, some differentiation of tissues can be made even by limited MR techniques. As the field progresses, more accurate parameter determinations are expected. Spectroscopy promises the possibility of highly specific tissue information.[78,79]

Bone Tumors

Round cell tumors (Fig. 9-9) typically involve the marrow cavity and have a much lower signal than fat on T_1-weighted images, a lower signal than fat on N(H)-weighted images, and a much higher signal than fat on highly T_2-weighted images. Many other lesions including hemangiomas, many sarcomas, and most metastases can have similar signal intensities.[11-13]

Bone cysts typically have a lower signal on T_1-weighted images than the group of lesions discussed above, but this appearance is highly dependent upon the protein content of the fluid. Bone cysts can be very difficult to visualize on N(H)-weighted images. Cystic fluid usually has very high signal on T_2-weighted images. The anatomic appearance of a benign lesion (a well-defined sclerotic margin) is also seen by MR.

Osteoid matrix has low signal on T_1-, N(H)-, and T_2- weighted images. Therefore, most osteosarcomas (Fig. 9-10) and osteoid osteomas (Fig. 9-11) will have similar signal appearances. However, portions of these tumors may

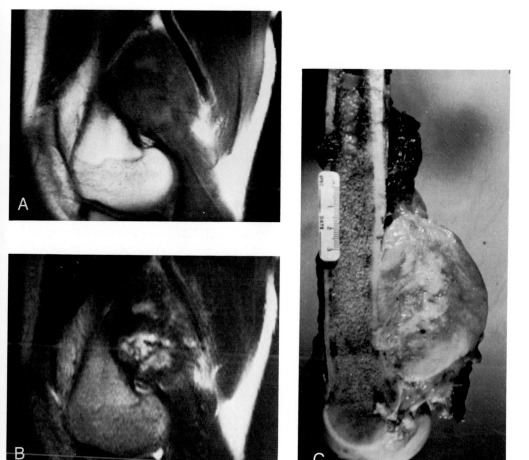

FIG. 9-7. Parosteal osteosarcoma. The (A) T_1- (TE 30, TR 500) and (B) T_2-weighted (TE 120, TR 2000) sagittal images of this poorly differentiated parosteal osteosarcoma demonstrate the ability of MR to define the extent of disease by delineating the vascular and bony anatomy. The (C) pathologic specimen is shown for correlation. A 2DFT multislice acquisition using a 5-inch diameter surface coil was employed for this scan.

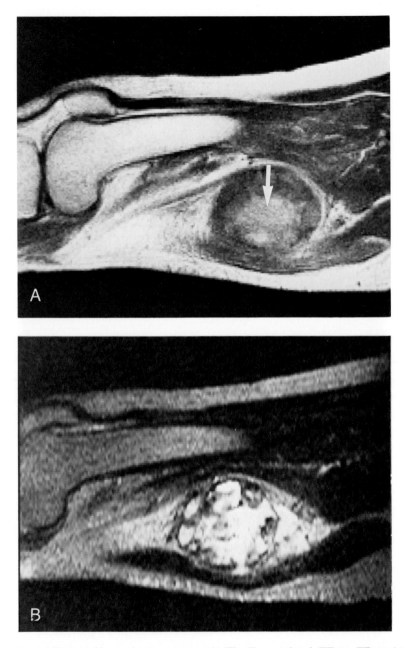

FIG. 9-8. Malignant fibrous histiocytoma. (A) The T_1-weighted (TE 30, TR 500) image shows a well defined soft tissue mass with an area of central necrosis (arrow). (B) The T_2-weighted (TE 120, TR 2000) image demonstrates and inhomogeneous mixed high- and low-signal tumor mass with edema extending within the surrounding fascial plane. These images were made with a 2DFT multislice acquisition in the body coil.

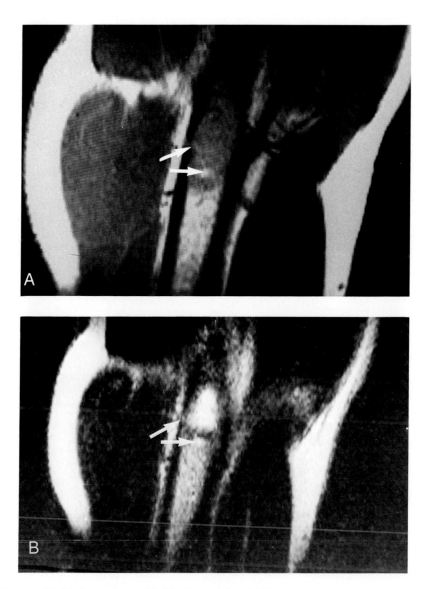

FIG. 9-9. Multiple myeloma. (A) The T_1-weighted (TE 30, TR 500) and (B) T_2-weighted (TE 120, TR 2000) images of the humerus show a homogeneous marrow-filling process with long T_1 (low signal) and T_2 (high signal) characteristics typical of a round cell tumor. A small area of high signal on the T_1- and T_2-weighted images (arrows) is blood in a pathologic fracture. These images utilized a 2DFT multislice acquisition and a saddle configuration surface coil.

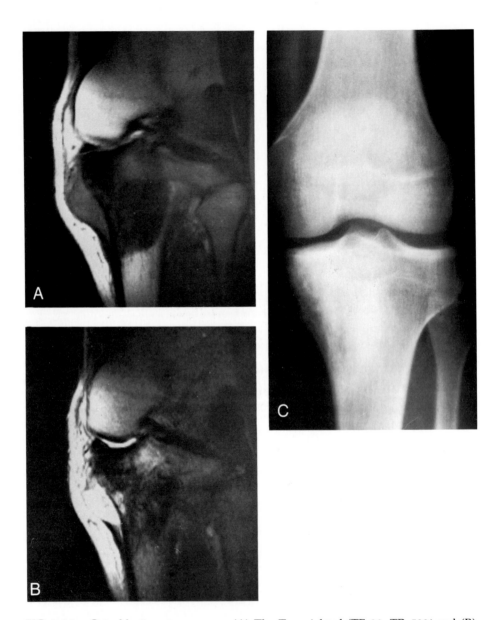

FIG. 9-10. Osteoblastic osteosarcoma. (A) The T_1-weighted (TE 30, TR 500) and (B) T_2-weighted (TE 120, TR 2000) coronal images of the proximal tibia show low signal from the osteoid matrix seen in the (C) radiograph. The tissue in the Codman's triangle has high signal on the T_2-weighted images. The MR images were obtained with a 2DFT multislice acquisition and a 5-inch diameter round surface coil.

FIG. 9-11. Osteoid osteoma. (A) The T_1-weighted (TE 30, TR 500), (B) T_2-weighted (TE 120, TR 2000), and (C) N(H)-weighted (TE 30, TR 1000) images of the distal fibula show low signal from the dense osteoid matrix on both images but higher signal from the nidus (arrow). A 2DFT multislice acquisition was used with a 5-inch diameter round surface coil for these images.

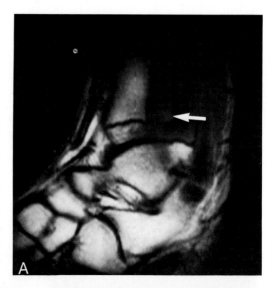

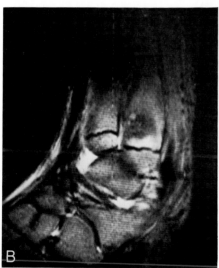

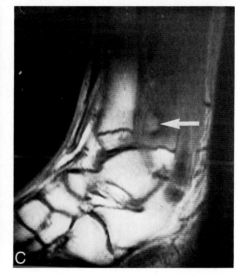

have other signal appearances. Because of the high chondroid tissue content, a chondroblastic osteosarcoma can have high signal on T_2-weighted images. Telangiectatic osteosarcoma (Fig. 9-12) has high signal on both T_1- and T_2-weighted images due to small hemorrhages.

Aneurysmal bone cyst (Fig. 9-13) is predominantly low signal on T_1- and T_2-weighted images with cystic areas of hemorrhage (high signal on both T_1- and T_2-weighted images).[80,81] Giant cell tumors have low signal on both T_1- and T_2-weighted images, reflecting the solid component of this lesion.[73]

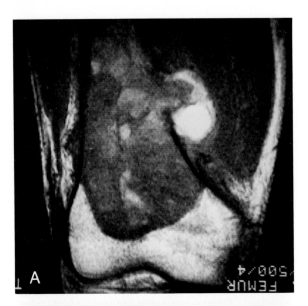

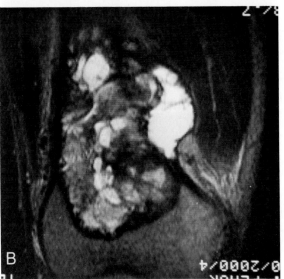

FIG. 9-12. Telangetatic osteosarcoma. (A) The T_1-weighted (TE 30, TR 500) image shows mixed high and low signal from the bone tumor. (B) The T_2-weighted (TE 120, TR 2000) image shows a similar pattern of mixed high and low signal. The hemorrhagic component of the mass has high signal on both the T_1- and T_2-weighted images. The osteoid matrix has low signal on both T_1- and T_2-weighted images. These images were performed with a 2DFT multislice acquisition and a 5-inch² surface coil.

Rarely, giant cell tumors can have large cystic components (Fig. 9-14) similar to aneurysmal bone cysts.

Chondroid tumors have mixed signal appearances. The characteristics of fat, bone, and chondroid matrix are seen in osteochondromas. Chondrosarcomas have varying amounts of high signal chondroid matrix on T_2-weighted images. The thickness of the cartilage cap can be directly measured by MR as a possible indicator of tumor malignancy.

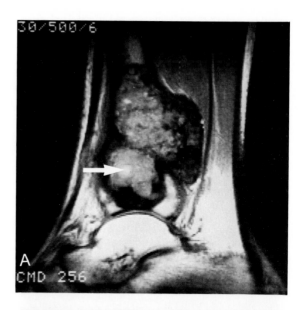

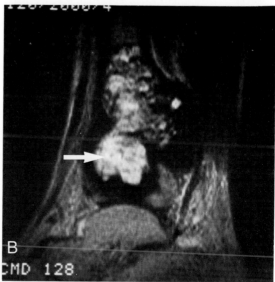

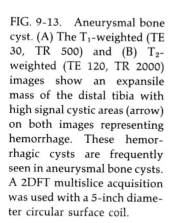

FIG. 9-13. Aneurysmal bone cyst. (A) The T_1-weighted (TE 30, TR 500) and (B) T_2-weighted (TE 120, TR 2000) images show an expansile mass of the distal tibia with high signal cystic areas (arrow) on both images representing hemorrhage. These hemorrhagic cysts are frequently seen in aneurysmal bone cysts. A 2DFT multislice acquisition was used with a 5-inch diameter circular surface coil.

Soft Tissue Tumors

Flowing blood usually results in a signal void. Arteriovenous malformations typically have low signal on both T_1- and T_2-weighted images (Fig. 9-15). The appearance of tubular or serpiginous structures of low signal intensity is characteristic. Lesions with high fat content including lipomas (Fig. 9-16) dermoids, and well-differentiated liposarcomas have high signal on T_1-weighted

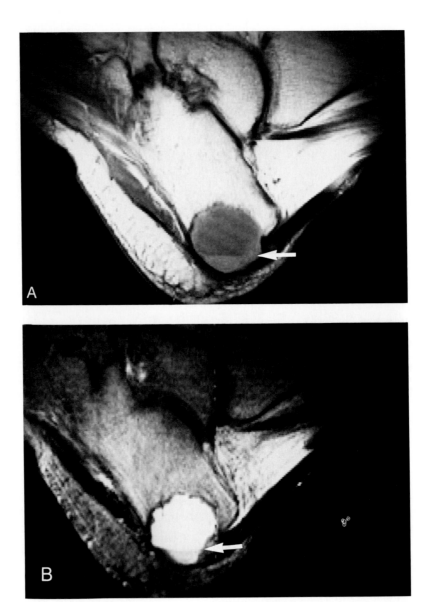

FIG. 9-14. Cystic giant cell tumor. (A) The T_1-weighted (TE 30, TR 500) and (B) T_2-weighted (TE 120, TR 2000) sagittal images of the calcaneus demonstrate a cystic mass with a fluid-fluid level (arrows) that could not be seen by CT. These images were made with a 2DFT multislice acquisition using a 5-inch diameter circular surface coil.

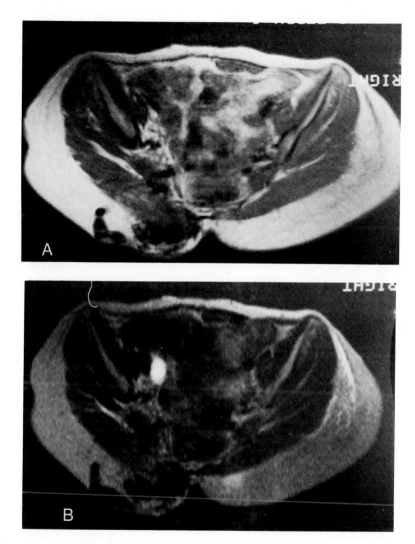

FIG. 9-15.   A large arteriovenous malformation of the hip is seen as a number of serpiginous channels of low signal on both (A) the T_1-weighted (TE 30, TR 500) and (B) T_2-weighted (TE 120, TR 2000) images. The extent of the lesion and definition of the feeding vessels are well defined by MR. These images were made with a 2DFT multislice acquisition in the body coil.

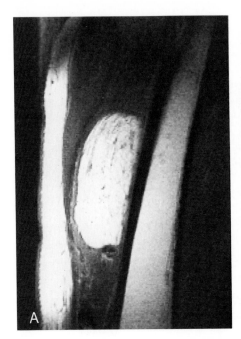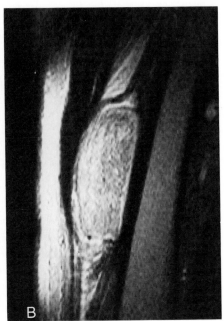

FIG. 9-16. Lipoma. (A) The T_1-weighted (TE 30, TR 500) image shows high signal from the well-defined intramuscular lipoma due to the short T_1 of fat (B) The T_2-weighted (TE 120, TR 2000) demonstrates a moderate signal intensity mass. Because of the short T_2 of fat, lipomas do not have high signal on T_2-weighted images. Heavy T_2 weighting is needed to demonstrate this effect. Some early papers even stated that fat had high signal on T_2-weighted images because the TE was not sufficiently long to show the short T_2 effect. A 2DFT multislice acquisition was used with a saddle-shaped surface coil for these images.

images, moderately high signal on N(H)-weighted images, and moderate signal on T_2-weighted images. At this time, a well-differentiated liposarcoma cannot be reliably distinguished from a lipoma. Poorly differentiated liposarcomas, however, usually are similar in signal to most other sarcomas.

Subacute hemorrhage has high signal on both T_1- and T_2- weighted images. Over time the signal within the central portion of the hematoma decreases. The other lesions with these signal appearances are quite limited. Only highly proteinaceous fluids or mucus have high intensity on both T_1- and T_2-weighted images. These lesions, however, do not typically have central low signal.

Most soft tissue sarcomas and histiocytomas have moderate signal on T_1-weighted images but a bizarre mixed high and low signal on T_2-weighted images (Fig. 9-8).[9,10,76,82] Areas of hemorrhage or necrosis can frequently be seen. Some malignant tumors, however, can be very homogeneous (Fig. 9-17). The presence of adjacent soft tissue edema may also be present in highly

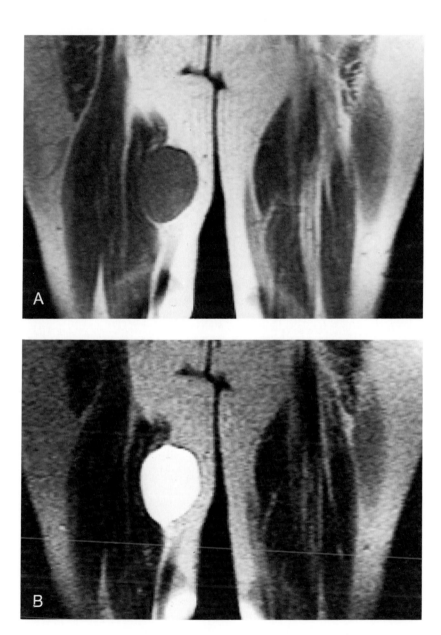

FIG. 9-17. This poorly differentiated liposarcoma has homogeneous moderate signal on (A) the T_1-weighted (TE 30, TR 500) image, but high signal on (B) the T_2-weighted (TE 120, TR 2000) image. Well-differentiated liposarcomas can be difficult to distinguish from a benign lipoma (Fig. 9-16). These images were made with a 2DFT multislice acquisition in the body coil.

aggressive lesions. Most melanomas have moderate signal on T_1-weighted images and relatively higher signal on T_2-weighted images.

Benign tumors in general are more homogeneous. This factor, however, cannot be used to differentiate benign from malignant since several malignant tumors have been homogeneous and vice versa. Hemangiomas (Fig. 9-18) are usually very homogeneous with moderate signal on T_1-weighted images and very high signal on T_2-weighted images. Neurofibromas can be either homogeneous or mixed (Fig. 9-19). The lack of soft tissue edema is a sign of a less aggressive tumor.[9-12]

Infection

In the treatment of musculoskeletal infections it is important to know the tissues involved by the infectious process. An osteomyelitis is treated much more aggressively than a cellulitis. Inadequate treatment of septic joints can lead to severe long-term complications. Bone scans often cannot differentiate these processes. Radiographs lack the sensitivity needed to identify many early infections. Early evidence indicates that MR is probably the most sensitive and specific method for evaluating this group of diseases.[82,83]

As described previously, normal marrow fat has high signal on T_1-weighted images and low signal on T_2-weighted images. In osteomyelitis (Fig. 9-20) the marrow has low signal on T_1-weighted images and high signal on T_2-weighted images. A normal marrow signal makes osteomyelitis an unlikely diagnosis.

High signal can be seen in the soft tissues affected by cellulitis (Fig. 9-21) or abscess. The extent of soft tissue involvement by the infectious process can be determined by MR in the absence of a defined mass effect. MR is, therefore, favored over CT in the evaluation of soft tissue infections and compartment syndromes.

Osteonecrosis

MR is a highly sensitive method for determining alterations in the bone marrow. A number of studies now indicate a significant diagnostic role for MR in the evaluation of osteonecrosis.[84,85] Osteonecrosis (Fig. 9-22) results in a decreased marrow signal on T_1-weighted images, usually in a vascular distribution. The appearance of osteonecrosis on T_2-weighted images depends upon the age of the lesion, surrounding edema, subsequent fractures, or hemorrhage.

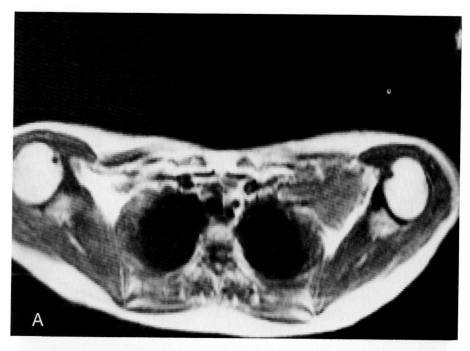

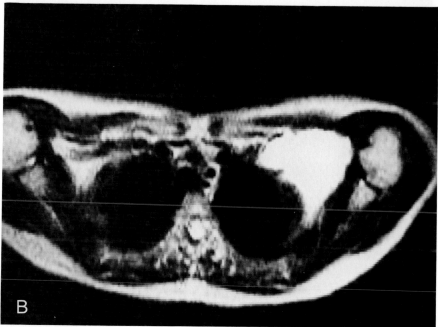

FIG. 9-18.   Hemangiomas typically have homogeneous moderate signal on (A) T_1-weighted (TE 30, TR 500) and high signal on (B) T_2-weighted (TE 120, TR 2000) images. A 2DFT multislice acquisition was used in the body coil.

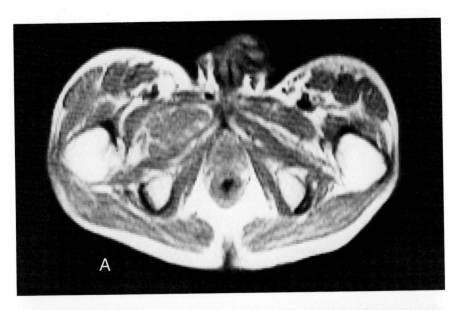

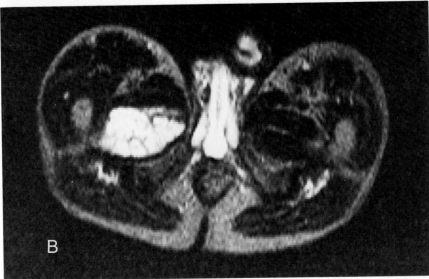

FIG. 9-19.   Neurofibroma. (A) The T_1-weighted (TE 30, TR 500) image shows an inhomogeneous but well-defined moderate signal mass. (B) The T_2-weighted (TE 120, TR 2000) image shows a well-defined, high signal mass with no surrounding edema. In another patient with neurofibromatosis, the pelvic neurofibromas are well seen on (C) the T_1-weighted (TE 30, TR 500) and (D) T_2-weighted (TE 120, TR 2000) exams. These images were made with a 2DFT multislice acquisition in the body coil.

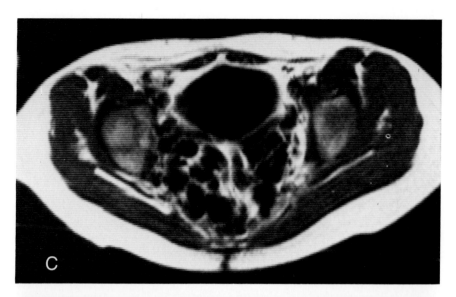

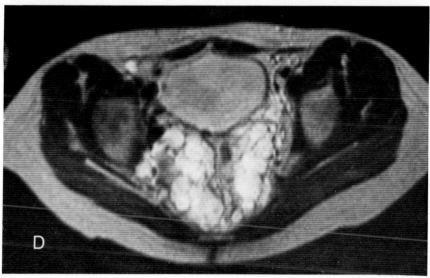

FIG. 9-19. (*continued*).

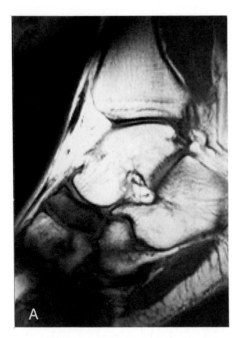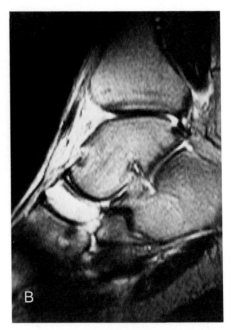

FIG. 9-20. Osteomyelitis. (A) The T_1-weighted (TE 30, TR 500) image shows low signal from the marrow of the navicular compared to the typical high-signal marrow fat seen in the other bones. (B) The T_2-weighted image demonstrates homogeneous high signal from the marrow of the navicular. This patient had markedly increased uptake on the radionuclide bone scan. The radiographs and CT scan were interpreted as normal except for soft tissue swelling. The MR clearly identifies the marrow disease as evidence of osteomyelitis. A saddle-shaped surface coil and a 2DFT multislice acquisition were used to generate the images.

Joint Disease

Magnetic resonance imaging has been used in the evaluation of the wrist, knee,[86-89] and temporomandibular joints.[90-91] In the wrist, MRI can be used to evaluate the carpal bones for evidence of osteonecrosis. The triangular cartilage can be directly visualized (Fig. 9-23). The intercarpal ligaments could also be evaluated by MRI, as can tears of the ligaments and menisci (Fig. 9-24) of the knee.[86,87] The soft tissue structures of the knee are directly visualized by MRI.

The clinical value of MRI for evaluating knee injuries is difficult to determine relative to arthroscopy. MRI may be most useful in evaluating knee injuries that are non-surgical in nature. A reliable, sensitive, and noninvasive test could have a significant role in evaluating these abnormalities.

To improve the sensitivity of MRI for small injuries of the knee, the thin-slice, selective 3D acquisition was developed.[89-92] Slices ranging from 0.6 to

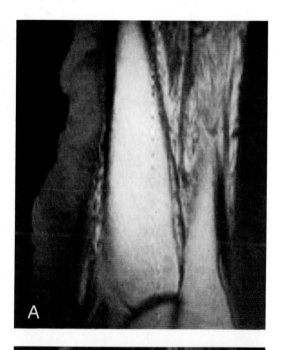

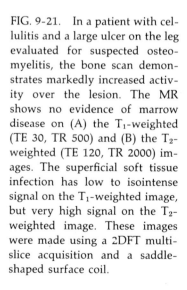

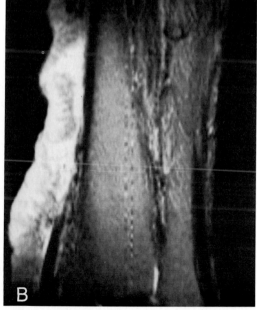

FIG. 9-21. In a patient with cellulitis and a large ulcer on the leg evaluated for suspected osteomyelitis, the bone scan demonstrates markedly increased activity over the lesion. The MR shows no evidence of marrow disease on (A) the T_1-weighted (TE 30, TR 500) and (B) the T_2-weighted (TE 120, TR 2000) images. The superficial soft tissue infection has low to isointense signal on the T_1-weighted image, but very high signal on the T_2-weighted image. These images were made using a 2DFT multi-slice acquisition and a saddle-shaped surface coil.

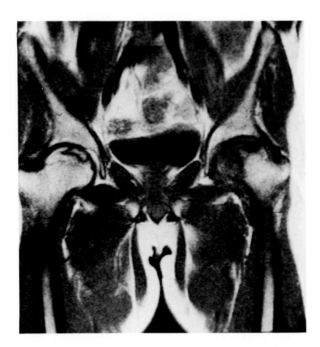

FIG. 9-22. Osteonecrosis. A T_1-weighted (TE 24, TR 500) image shows low signal from the marrow fat and flattening of the articular surface of the left hip due to osteonecrosis. This image was made in the body coil using a 2DFT multislice acquisition.

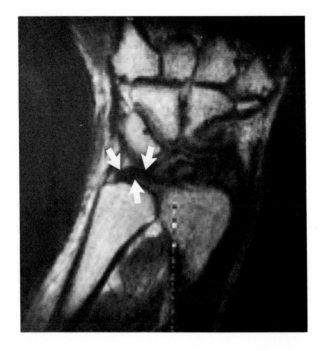

FIG. 9-23. Normal wrist. The bony and soft tissue anatomy are well seen on this thin-slice (1-mm) selective 3D image of the triangular cartilage (arrows).

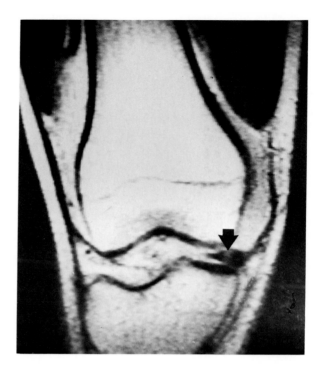

FIG. 9-24. A tear of the meniscus is seen on this T_1-weighted (TE 30, TR 500) image (arrow). A round, 5-inch diameter flat surface coil combined with a 2DFT multislice acquisition was employed for a set of 5-mm thick slices with 20 percent gaps between slices.

1 mm are acquired. Using this method, anatomic detail is expected to be sufficient to visualize very small tears (Fig. 9-25).

The temporomandibular joint (TMJ) is well suited for MRI evaluation, and MRI is likely to become the method of choice for evaluating most TMJ disorders.[90-92] The proximity to the skin surface is excellent for surface coil positioning. The accurate assessment of the disc is important in the clinical diagnosis and management. The disc and associated soft tissue structures can be directly visualized by MRI without the use of contrast agents.

SUMMARY

The greatest advantage of MRI at present is its ability to determine the extent of disease accurately. In many cases, the anatomic appearance along with the clinical setting can define a good differential. As our knowledge of MR improves, the MR signal characteristics could improve the specificity of the exam. An outline of the signal appearances that have appeared with certain lesions are outlined in Table 9-2.

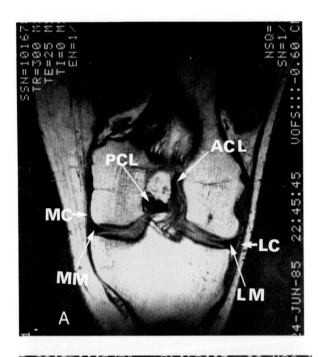

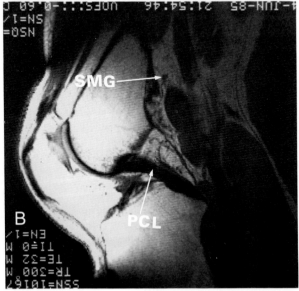

FIG. 9-25. High-resolution images of the knee. A selective 3DFT acquisition combined with a saddle-shaped surface coil produced these T_1-weighted (TE 26, TR 300) 0.8 mm thick slices. Examples of (A) coronal and (B) sagittal images are shown. The superior medial geniculate artery (SMG) posterior cruciate ligament (PCL), anterior cruciate ligament (ACL), medial collateral ligament (MC), lateral collateral ligament (LC), medial meniscus (MM), and lateral meniscus (LM) are labeled.

TABLE 9-2. Tissue signal patterns on MRI

High signal T_1-weighted, high signal T_2-weighted
  Hemorrhage (subacute)
  Proteinaceous fluids
  Necrosis
  Mucus-containing cysts
High signal T_1-weighted, low signal T_2-weighted
  Lipoma
  Well-differentiated liposarcoma
  Melanoma
Low signal T_1-weighted, high signal T_2-weighted
  Hemorrhage (acute)
  Most metastases
  Lymphoma
  Leukemia
  Most soft tissue sarcomas
  Neurofibroma
  Most cysts
  Infarction
  Round cell tumor
  Hemangioma
  Malignant fibrous histiocytoma
  Melanoma
  Chondroblastic osteosarcoma
Low signal T_1-weighted, low signal T_2-weighted
  Osteosarcoma (osteoid matrix)
  Giant cell tumor
  Aneurysmal bone cyst
  Fibrous dysplasia
  Fibrous cortical defect
  Osteofibrous dysplasia
  Myelofibrosis
  Sickle cell (except infarcts)
  Osteoid osteoma
  Osteoblastoma
  Arteriovenous malformation
  Osteonecrosis
Low signal T_1-weighted, mixed low and high signal T_2-weighted
  Osteochondroma
  Enchondroma
  Chondrosarcoma
  Osteonecrosis (early)
  Osteosarcoma (mixed cellularity)
  Many soft tissue sarcomas and histiocytomas

FUTURE ADVANCES

MR applications are expected to advance rapidly both in the clinical area and technologically. The development of fast scan methods could provide near real-time imaging capability and improved efficiency.[70-72] Since MR detects lesions missed by other modalities, MR biopsy needles are being developed to take advantage of the increased sensitivity. Specialized receiver coils are being designed to improve resolution dramatically.[56-62] Contrast agents are being investigated not only as a complement to currently used radiologic[93,94] methods but also as specific probes of tissue physiology.[95,96] Spectroscopy is being intensely investigated for the wealth of biochemical data available from tissue spectra.[78,79,97] Nuclei other than hydrogen are being explored: ^{23}Na imaging can yield specific information on the Na-K pump and tissue energy metabolism,[98,99] and ^{19}F-labeled agents could be used for vascular contrast or as a tracer.[100,101] Three-dimensional displays are being developed to make better use of volume acquisition data.[102-104] As the clinical achievements of MR becomes apparent, the encouragement for technologic advancement will accelerate.

CONCLUSION

In a relatively short period of clinical use, MRI has become a major diagnostic method in the evaluation of musculoskeletal disorders. Its lack of biologic hazards[105-110] is important to most patients. The soft tissue anatomy of MR surpasses most conventional techniques and often MR can provide improved lesion specificity. As clinical knowledge increases, MR could replace other imaging methods for the evaluation of many musculoskeletal conditions.

MR does have some significant limitations: the equipment is expensive and difficult to site, and the technology is complex and foreign to many medical personnel. These factors contribute to delayed implementation and acceptance of MR.

While many of the current limitations of MR will improve with time, perhaps the greatest challenge of the future will be the ability of practitioners to maintain a working knowledge of this rapidly changing technology.

REFERENCES

1. Smith FW: Whole body nuclear magnetic resonance imaging. Radiography 47:297, 1981
2. Young IR, Bailes DR, Burl M et al: Initial clinical evaluation of a whole body nuclear magnetic resonance (NMR) tomograph. J Comput Assist Tomogr 6:1, 1982
3. Crooks L, Arakawa M, Hoenninger J et al: Nuclear magnetic resonance whole-body imager operating at 3.5 Kgauss. Radiology 143:169, 1982
4. Alfidi RJ, Haaga JR, El Yousef SJ et al: Preliminary experimental results in humans and animals with a superconducting, whole-body, nuclear magnetic resonance scanner. Radiology 143:175, 1982
5. Worthington BS: Clinical prospects for nuclear magnetic resonance. Clin Radiol 34:3, 1983

6. Steiner RE: The Hammersmith experience with nuclear magnetic resonance. Clin Radiol 34:13, 1983

7. Smith FW: Two years clinical experience with NMR imaging. Appl Radiol May/June:29–42, 1983

8. Bottomley PA, Edelstein WA, Leue WM et al: Head and body imaging by hydrogen nuclear magnetic resonance. Magn Reson Imaging 1:69, 1982

9. Moon KL, Jr. Genant KH, Helms CA et al: Musculoskeletal applications of nuclear magnetic resonance. Radiology 147:161, 1983

10. Berquist TH: Magnetic resonance imaging: preliminary experience in orthopedic radiology. Magn Reson Imaging 2:41, 1984

11. Harms SE: Three dimensional imaging of bone and joint pathology. Program, Society of Magnetic Resonance in Medicine 302–303, 1984

12. Fenstermacher MJ, Harms SE, Greenway GD: Optimization of MR techniques for the diagnosis of bone and joint diseases. Radiology 153:116, 1984

13. Zimmer WD, Berquist TH, McLeod RA et al: Bone tumors: magnetic resonance imaging versus computed tomography. Radiology 155:709, 1985.

14. Harms SE, Morgan TJ, Yamanashi WS et al: Principles of nuclear magnetic resonance imaging. Radiographics 4:26, 1984

15. Harms SE, Kramer DM: Fundamentals of magnetic resonance imaging. CRC Crit Rev Diagn Imag 25:79, 1985

16. Fullerton GD: Basic concepts for nuclear magnetic resonance imaging. Magn Reson Imaging 1:39, 1982

17. Hoult DI: An overview of NMR in medicine. National Center for Health Care Technology, HEW, 1981

18. Rosen BR, Brady TJ: Principles of nuclear magnetic resonance for medical applications. Sem in Nucl Med 13:308, 1984

19. Pykett IL: NMR imaging in medicine. Sci Am 246:78, 1982

20. Pykett IL, Newhouse JH, Buonanno FS et al: Principles of nuclear magnetic resonance imaging. Radiology 143:157, 1982

21. Kramer DM: Basic principles of magnetic resonance imaging. Radiol Clin North Am 22:765, 1984

22. Petersen SB, Muller RN, Rinck PA: An Introduction to Biomedical Nuclear Magnetic Resonance. Thieme-Stratton, New York, 1985

23. Fukushima E, Roeder SBW: Experimental Pulse NMR: A Nuts and Bolts Approach. Addison-Wesley, Reading, 1981

24. Mansfield P, Morris PG: NMR Imaging in Biomedicine. Academic Press, New York, 1982

25. Gudian DG: Nuclear Magnetic Resonance and Its Applications to Living Sytems. Clarendon Press, New York, 1982

26. Partain CL, James AE, Rollo FD et al: Nuclear Magnetic Resonance Imaging. WB Saunders, Philadelphia, 1983

27. Axel L (ed): Glossary of Nuclear Magnetic Resonance (NMR) Terms. American College of Radiology, Bethesda, 1983

28. Singer JR: Blood-flow rates by NMR measurements. Science 130:1652, 1959

29. Hemminga MA, DeJuger PA: The study of flow by pulsed nuclear magnetic resonance II. Measurement of flow velocities using a repetitive pulse method. J Magn Reson 37:1, 1980

30. Kaufman L, Crooks LE, Sheldon PE et al: Evaluation of NMR imaging for detection and quantification of obstructions in vessels. Invest Radiol 17:554, 1982

31. Hemminga MA: Measurement of flow characteristics using nuclear magnetic resonance. p. 157. In James TL, Margulis AR (eds): Biomedical Magnetic Resonance. Radiology Research and Education Foundation, San Francisco, 1984

32. Moran PR: A flow velocity zeugmatographic interface for NMR imaging in humans. Magn Reson Imaging 1:197, 1983

33. Wesby GE, Moseley ME, Ehman RL: Translational molecular self-diffusion in magnetic resonance imaging I. Effects on observed spin-spin relaxation. Invest Radiol 19:484, 1984

34. Wesby GE, Moseley ME, Ehman RL: Translational molecular self-diffusion in magnetic resonance imaging II. Measurement of the self-diffusion coefficient. Invest Radiol 19:491, 1984

35. Dixon WT: Simple proton spectroscopic imaging. Radiology 153:184, 1984

36. Brown TR, Kincaid BM, Ugurbil K: NMR chemical shift imaging in three dimensions. Proc Natl Acad Sci USA 79:3523, 1982

37. Joseph PM: A spin echo chemical shift MR imaging technique. J Comput Assist Tomogr 9:651, 1985

38. Kaplan JI, Frankel G: NMR of Chemically Exchanging Systems. Academic Press, New York, 1980

39. James TL: Nuclear Magnetic Resonance in Biochemistry. Academic Press, New York, 1975

40. Jarcletzky O, Roberts GCK: NMR in Molecular Biology. Academic Press, New York, 1981

41. Dwek RA: Nuclear Magnetic Resonance in Biochemistry: Application to Enzyme systems. Clarendon Press, Oxford, 1973

42. Bryant RG: Water proton relaxation. p. 127. In James TL, Margulis AR (eds): Biomedical Magnetic Resonance Imaging. Radiology Research and Education Foundation, San Francisco, 1984

43. Foster MA: Magnetic Resonance in Medicine and Biology. Pergamon Press, Oxford, 1984

44. Clegg JS: Metabolism and the intracellular environment: the vicinal water network model. p. 363. In Drost-Hansen W, Clegg JS (eds): Cell-Associated Water. Academic Press, New York, 1979

45. Packer KJ: The dynamics of water in heterogeneous systems. Phil Trans R Soc Lond B 278:59, 1977

46. Ling GN: The physical state of water in living cells and its physiological significance. Int J Neurosci 1:129, 1970

47. Hazlewood CF: A view of the significance and understanding of the physical properties of cell-associated water. p. 165. In Drost-Hansen W, Clegg JS (eds): Cell-Associated Water. Academic Press, New York, 1979

48. Damadian R: Tumor detection by nuclear magnetic resonance. Science 171:1151, 1971

49. Eggleston JC, Saryan LA, Hollis DP: Nuclear magnetic resonance investigations of human neoplastic and abnormal non-neoplastic tissues. Cancer Res 35:1326, 1975

50. Koivula A, Kauppila A, Kiviniitty K et al: Investigation of gynecological cancer with nuclear magnetic relaxation methods. Strablentherapie 149:402, 1975

51. Fruchter RG, Goldsmith M, Boyce JG et al: Nuclear magnetic resonance properties of gynecological tissues. Gynecol Oncol 6:242, 1978

52. Schara M, Sentijure M, Auersperg M, Golouh R: Characterization of malignant thyroid gland tissue by magnetic resonance methods. Br J Cancer 29:483, 1974

53. Lauterbur PC: Image formatin by induced local interaction: examples employing nuclear magnetic resonance. Nature 242:190, 1973

54. Beall PT, Amtey SR, Kastari SR: NMR Data Handbook for Biomedical Applications. Pergamon Press, New York, 1984

55. Davis PL, Kaufman L, Crooks LE: Tissue characterization, p. 53. In Margulis AR, Higgins CB, Kaufman L, Crooks LE (eds): Clinical Magnetic Resonance Imaging. San Francisco, Radiology Research and Education Foundation, 1983

56. El Yousef SJ, Duchesneau RH, Alfidi RJ: Nuclear magnetic resonance imaging of the breast. Radiographics 4:113, 1984

57. Alcorn FS, Turner DA, Clark JW et al: Magnetic resonance imaging in the study of the breast. Radiographics 5:631, 1985

58. Ng TC, Glickson JD: Shielded solenoidal probe for in vivo NMR studies of solid tumors. Magn Reson Med 2:169, 1985

59. Fitzsimmons JR, Thomas RG, Mancuso AA: Proton imaging with surface coils on a 0.15-T resistive system. Magn Reson Med 2:180, 1985

60. Bydder GM, Curati WL, Gadian DG et al: Use of closely coupled receiver coils in MR imaging: practical aspects. J Comput Assist Tomogr 9:987, 1985

61. Gallimore GW, Jr., Harms SE: High resolution MR imaging of knee injuries. Radiology 157:275, 1985

62. Lufkin RB, Hanafee W: Application of surface coils to NMR anatomy of the larynx. AJNR 6:491, 1985

63. National Radiological Protection Board: Advice on acceptable limits of exposure to nuclear magnetic resonance clinical imaging. Radiography 50:221, 1984

64. Harms, SE, Siemers PT, Hildenbrand P, Plum G: Multiple spin echo magnetic resonance imaging of the brain. Radiographics 6(1):117, 1986

65. Harms SE: Three dimensional multiple echo imaging of human brain pathology. Program, Third Annual Meeting Society of Magnetic Resonance in Medicine p. 304–305, 1984

66. Garroway AN, Grannell PK, Mansfield P: Image formation in NMR by a selective irradiative process. J Phys [C] 7:457, 1974

67. Crooks LE, Ortendahl DA, Kaufman L et al: Clinical efficiency of nuclear magnetic resonance imaging. Radiology 146:123, 1983

68. Kumar A, Welti D, Ernst R: NMR Fourier zeugmatography. J Magn Reson 18:69, 1975

69. Kramer DM, Compton RA, Yeung HN: A volume (3D) analogue of 2D multislice or "multislab" MR imaging. Program, Fourth Annual Meeting Society of Magnetic Resonance in Medicine 162–163, 1985

70. Mansfield P, Redzian RR, Doyle M et al: Real-time echo-planar imaging in pediatrics. J Magn Reson Med 1:125, 1984

71. Haaske EM, Clayton JR, Linga NR, Bearden FH: Demonstration of a flexible fast scan technique. Radiology 153:244, 1984

72. Mansfield P, Doyle M, Chapman B et al: Real time proton imaging of the heart: some clinical results. Program, Fourth Annual Meeting Society of Magnetic Resonance in Medicine, 631–632, 1985

73. Brady TJ, Gebhardt MC, Pykett IL et al: NMR imaging of forearms in healthy volunteers and patients with giant-cell tumors of bone. Radiology 144:549, 1982

74. Cohen MD, Klatte EC, Baehner R et al: Magnetic resonance imaging of the bone marrow disease in children. Radiology 151:715, 1984

75. Brady TJ, Rosen BR, Pykett IL et al: NMR imaging of leg tumors. Radiology 149:181, 1983

76. Seeger LL, Bassett L, Bertino F, Hanafee W: Magnetic resonance imaging for demonstrating undetected bone metastases. General Program, 16th International Congress of Radiology 1985, p. 137

77. Kaufman L, Crooks LE, Sheldon PE et al: The potential impact of nuclear magnetic resonance on cardiovascular diagnosis. Circulation 67:251, 1983

78. James TL, Margulis AR (eds): Biomedical Magnetic Resonance. Radiology Research and Education Foundation, San Francisco, 1984

79. Newman RJ: Clinical applications of nuclear magnetic resonance spectroscopy: a review. J R Soc Med 77:774, 1984

80. Zimmer WD, Berquist TH, Sim FH et al: Magnetic resonance imaging of aneurysmal bone cyst. Mayo Clin Proc 59:633, 1984

81. Hudson TM, Hamlin DJ, Fitzsimmons JR: Magnetic resonance imaging of fluid levels in an aneurysmal bone cyst and in anticoagulated human blood. Skel Radiol 13:267, 1985

82. Ross RJ, Thompson JS, Kim K, Bailey R: Nuclear magnetic resonance evaluation of a leiomyosarcoma. Magn Reson Imaging 1:87, 1982

83. Fletcher BD, Scoles PV, Nelson AD: Osteomyelitis in children: detection by magnetic resonance. Radiology 150:57, 1984

84. Totty WG, Murphy WA, Ganz WI et al: Magnetic resonance imaging of the normal and ischemic femoral head. AJR 143:1273–1280, 1984

85. Brasch RC, Wesby GE, Gooding CA et al: Magnetic resonance imaging of transfusional hemosiderosis complicating thalessemia major. Radiology 150:767, 1984

86. Li KC, Henkelman M, Poon PY, Rubenstein J: MR imaging of the normal knee. J Comput Assist Tomogr 8:1147, 1985

87. Kean DM, Worthington BS, Preston BJ et al: Nuclear magnetic resonance imaging of the knee: examples of normal anatomy and pathology. Br J Radiol 56:355, 1983

88. Turner DA, Prodromos CC, Petasnick JP, Clark JW: Acute injury of the ligaments of the knee: magnetic resonance evaluation. Radiology 154:717, 1985

89. Muschler G, Cohen J, Harms S et al: Normal and pathologic knee anatomy with correlation of anatomic disection and chemical differences of collagenous and collagen-mineral tissues from fresh cadaver specimens. Program, Fourth Annual Meeting Society of Magnetic Resonance in Medicine, 1184–1185, 1985

90. Harms SE, Wilk RM, Wolford LM et al: The temporomandibular joint: magnetic resonance imaging using surface coils. Radiology 157:133, 1985

91. Roberts D, Schenck J, Joseph P et al: Temporomandibular joint imaging. Radiology 155:829, 1985

92. Harms SE, Kramer DM: Selective three-dimensional imaging of neurological disease using a surface coil. Program, Fourth Annual Meeting Society of Magnetic Resonance in Medicine, pp. 359–360, 1985

93. Carr DH, Brown GM, Bydder GM et al: Gadolinium-DTPA as a contrast agent in MRI: initial clinical experience in 20 patients. AJR 143:215–224, 1984

94. Runge VM, Clanton JA, Price AC: Contrast enhanced magnetic resonance evaluation of a brain abscess model. AJNR 6:139–147, 1985

95. Patronas NJ, Knop RH, Hambright P et al: Paramagnetic labeled hematoporphyrin deriivitive (HPD) as a human tumor localizing agent for laser phototherapy directed treatment in MRI images. Program, Fourth Annual Meeting Society of Magnetic Resonance in Medicine, vol. 2, pp. 890–891, 1985

96. Swartz HM, Bennett RD, Brown RD: Feasibility of measuring redox metabolism by nitroxide contrast agents. Program, Fourth Annual Meeting Society of Magnetic Resonance in Medicine, vol. 2, pp. 834–835, 1985

97. Shulman GI, Alger JR, Prichard JW et al: Nuclear magnetic resonance spectroscopy in diagnostic and investigative medicine. J Clin Invest 109:430, 1984

98. Maudsley AA, Hilal SK: Biological aspects of ^{23}Na imaging. Br Med Bull 40:155, 1984

99. Hilal SK, Maudsley AA, Simon HE et al: In vivo NMR of sodium-23 in the human head. J Comput Assist Tomogr 9:1, 1985

100. Joseph PM, Fishman JE, Mukherji L et al: Vascular imaging in rats with ^{19}F MRI. Program, Fourth Annual Meeting Society of Magnetic Resonance in Medicine, vol. 2, pp. 995–996, 1985

101. Mcfarland E, Koutcher JA, Rosen BR et al: In vivo ^{19}F NMR imaging. J Comput Assist Tomogr 9:8, 1985

102. Herman GT: Three dimensional imaging from tomograms p. 93. In Hohne KH (ed): Digital Imaging Processing in Medicine. Springer-Verlag, Berlin, 1981

103. Axel L, Herman GT, Udupa JK et al: Three-dimensional display of nuclear magnetic resonance (NMR) cardiovascular images. J Comput Assist Tomogr 7:172, 1983

104. Herman GT: Three-dimensional display of organs based on magnetic resonance imaging. Program, Fourth Annual Meeting Society of Magnetic Resonance in Medicine, vol. 1, pp. 189–190, 1985

105. Budinger TF, Cullander C: Health effects of in vivo nuclear magnetic resonance. p. 421. In James TL, Margulis AR (eds): Biomedical Magnetic Resonance. Radiology Research and Education Foundation, San Francisco, 1984

106. Wolff S, James TL, Young GB: Magnetic resonance imaging: absence of in vitro cytogenic damage. Radiology 155:163, 1985

107. Budinger TF, Cullander C: Health hazards in nuclear magnetic resonance in vivo studies. Radiographics 4:74, 1984

108. Withers HR, Mason KA, Davis PA: MR effect on murine spermatogenesis. Radiology 156:741, 1985

109. Prasad N, Wright DA, Forster JD: Effect of nuclear magnetic resonance on early stages of amphibian development. Magn Reson Imaging 1:35, 1982

110. Prasad N, Bushong SC, Thornby JI et al: Effect of nuclear magnetic resonance on chromosomes of mouse bone marrow cells. Magn Reson Imaging 2:37, 1984

10 Advances in CT Imaging of Musculoskeletal Pathology

ELLIOT K. FISHMAN
DONNA MAGID
DOUGLAS D. ROBERTSON
BOB DREBIN
WILLIAM W. SCOTT, JR.

The development of computed body tomography has lead to revolutionary changes in the evaluation of musculoskeletal disorders. In the preceding chapters, the use of CT in the evaluation of both benign and malignant disease of the musculoskeletal system is discussed. The advantages and disadvantages of CT are carefully outlined.

However, we believe that advanced applications of CT in the evaluation of musculoskeletal disorders are just evolving. Recent interest in a more detailed, comprehensive, and systematic evaluation of the CT data has led major CT manufacturers to develop advanced software programs that are particularly helpful in the evaluation of the musculoskeletal system. These initial programs run on the main computers of the CT scanner and usually consist of two standard programs; the multiplanar reconstructions and display (MPR/MPD) and a variety of three-dimensional reconstruction programs. Recently several free-standing computer systems for the systematic evaluation of musculoskeletal disorders have been developed. Other more advanced systems are currently undergoing clinical trials. This chapter presents an overview of these programs, focusing on practical clinical applications. We also discuss the exciting area of using CT-generated data for the design of custom hip and knee implants. Finally, the use of real-time three-dimensional imaging with the Pixar system is discussed.

MULTIPLANAR RECONSTRUCTION

The potential usefulness of coronal and sagittal reformatted CT images was recognized soon after CT became available. By 1980 most manufacturers provided at least some capability to acquire selected reformatted images. Most centers, however, used these programs with little success and, at best, in selected cases.

In 1980, Dr. William Glenn and his associates showed that the evaluation of spinal pathology could be enhanced by presenting the data in sagittal and coronal formats in addition to the standard transaxial imaging program.[1,2] Dr. Glenn and his associates subsequently developed a sequential imaging program format marketed to other institutions by Multi-Planar Diagnostic Imaging, Inc., Torrance, California. Other manufacturers, including Siemens Medical Systems, developed similar MPR/D programs. Over the past 3 years we have used the MPR/D program on our Siemens DR-3 scanner for the evaluation of complex musculoskeletal pathologic change.[3,4] We have presently examined over 700 patients using the program and both the radiologists and orthopedic surgeons have found it to be very helpful. The areas where we have found the MPR/D program to be particularly helpful have been in acetabular trauma, the staging of avascular necrosis of the femoral head, and the evaluation of congenital hip disease.

The MPR/D program is user-friendly and easily adaptable to the evaluation of other types of pathology.

Specific Applications

The Hip

Our technique for evaluation of the hip is described here.[4] The patient is positioned supine, with the feet in the neutral anatomic position, and with knees and feet taped together to prevent inadvertent motion. Scanning begins at a level approximately 4 cm above the dome of the acetabulum. Consecutive 4-mm scans are obtained at 3-mm intervals through a level just below the lesser trochanter. This allows for a 1-mm overlap of images. The technical scanning factors are 3.2 sec, 230 mAs, 125 kVp, and 4-mm slice thickness. The usual number of scans obtained per patient is between 30 and 45. Following the acquisition of the transaxial images a specially designed software package is used for data manipulation. The package available on the Siemens DR-3 scanner is the multiplanar reconstruction and display software (MPR/D) (Siemens Medical Systems, Iselin, NJ).

The program automatically presents the middle transverse slice (of those requested) as a reference image. A reconstruction box is then chosen using a resister pen. The maximum area that can be reconstructed is 127 × 127 pixels. This would be sufficient to encompass the entire hemipelvis. Usually, however, a smaller area containing the appropriate anatomic area of interest is reconstructed. Interpolation of identical rows from each transaxial image creates a coronal view and interpolation of identical columns creates a sagittal view. During the reconstruction process, each coronal and sagittal view inside the defined box is produced and stored on the image disc. The total reconstruction time ranges between 2 and 10 minutes depending upon the number of sections obtained and on whether or not the scanner is being used to image additional patients simultaneously.

When the reconstruction is complete, several display modes are available. In the standard mode, a freely selectable reference transverse image is shown and single or multiple coronal or sagittal images can be obtained. The thickness of each view has a selectable width of 1 to 11 pixels. We have arbitrarily chosen a width of 3 pixels in all cases. A survey mode is available which will display every coronal and/or sagittal image. We routinely review and film every patient in the multiformat mode to obtain the most possible data. All image reconstructions are filmed using both muscle (WW-421, WC-36) and bone (WW-1000, WC-150 or WW-2000, WC-220) window width and level settings.

The two largest patient groups evaluated with the MPR/D program have been those with acetabular trauma and those with avascular necrosis of the femoral head.

Advantages

The advantages of CT/MPR in the assessment of the traumatized hip are covered in detail elsewhere (Chap. 4), but they include all the benefits of transaxial imaging (e.g., window manipulation to allow bone, joint space, and muscle compartment assessment; inclusion of the contralateral side to increase sensitivity to subtle change; detection of fractures poorly seen on plain roentgenograms) and also

1.   Definition of the key weight-bearing structures—the acetabular dome, the anterior and posterior columns, and the superior pole of the femur—on which the hip's stability and weight bearing support depend (Fig. 10-1).
2.   Assessment of the congruity and continuity of the joint surface.
3.   Detection of intra-articular fragments (bone or foreign matter).
4.   Definition of degree and direction of fragment displacement and rotation, and of column disruption.
5.   Confirming or characterizing the postoperative result, including both the immediate status of reduction and fixation and longer-term follow-up to assess healing, hardware problems, or complications such as nonunion or avascular necrosis.

Avascular Necrosis

Another major area where the CT findings have been enhanced with MPR/ D has been in the evaluation of avascular necrosis. The rising incidence of avascular necrosis of the femoral head (AVN) can be attributed in part to improved diagnostic methods but also reflects medical advances allowing the prolonged survival of the population at risk for nontraumatic AVN: patients with renal transplants, the immunosuppressed, those with collagen vascular

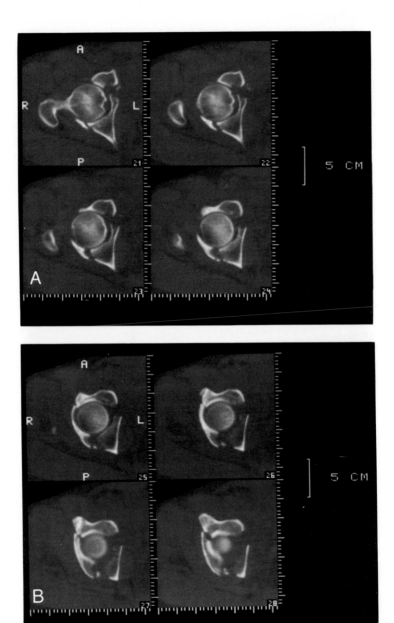

FIG. 10-1. In a 57-year-old man with T-type acetabular fracture, (A,B) transaxial images show fracture involving anterior and posterior acetabular columns and medial wall of acetabulum.

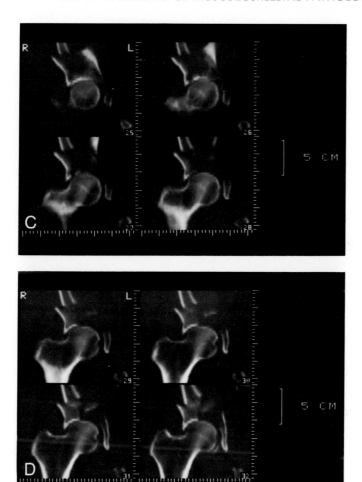

FIG. 10-1 (*continued*).   (C-F) Sequential coronal images demonstrate the full extent of disruption of the weight-bearing surface of the acetabulum.

disease, sickle cell disease, neoplasm, and others. This is a significantly younger group than those with traumatic AVN, and eventually 50 percent of this group will develop bilateral disease. Although there are differences in opinion as to the most effective treatment at each stage of disease, there is universal agreement that early diagnosis and intervention offer the only means of interrupting the relentless progressive destruction of the femoral head.[5-7]

Conventional radiography, the most common means of screening the patient with hip pain and of studying the patient with suspected AVN, may have a sensitivity to early disease as low as 41 percent.[8] When positive, plain films may underestimate the extent of disease, contour alteration, and acetabular involvement.

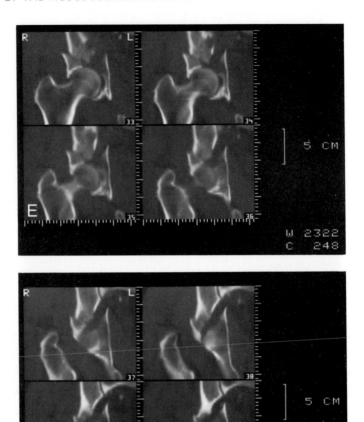

FIG. 10-1 (*continued*).

Computed tomography with multiplanar reconstructions (CT/MPR) has demonstrated its superiority over conventional radiography in the detection and staging of AVN.[3] Transaxial CT has superior sensitivity to subtle alterations of femoral head density and trabecular architecture, and CT/MPR allows demonstration of both normal and abnormal anatomy in three planes and without superimposition (Figs. 10-2 to 10-4).

A study designed to compare CT/MPR to conventional radiographic staging underlined the need to expand the current staging system. That system,[5] based on plain films, defines normal as stage 0, preradiographic but histologic disease as stage I, sclerotic and/or osteoporotic changes in an otherwise intact femoral head as stage II, contour alteration as stage III, and acetabular involvement as stage IV. We discovered that what had been called stage II and III was, in fact, a broad spectrum of disease. If therapeutic decisions were to be derived

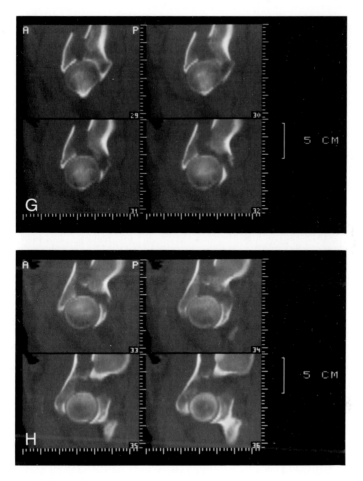

FIG. 10-1 (*continued*).   (G,H) Sequential sagittal views best demonstrate the relationship of the fracture to the joint space as well as the full extent of acetabular/roof disruption.

from and correlated to staging, further subdivision of these overly inclusive categories was necessary[3] (Table 10-1).

Transaxial CT using MPR technique yields several thin slices through the femoral head, allowing assessment of both contour and texture. Transaxial images through the midfemoral head transect the interdigitating tensile and compressive trabeculae, creating a characteristic honeycombed or "asterisk" appearance.[9] One of the earliest signs of AVN may be clumping or irregularity of this radial asterisk pattern, or coarsening of the regular texture of the head.[10] Where indicated, one or two 2-mm high-resolution images may be obtained to clarify suspected alterations. Transaxial images will also detect subchondral lucencies or undermining creating a "crescent sign." Subtle contour alteration may be detected far earlier than on plain film.

Even with thin slices, partial volume averaging limits transaxial visualization of the superior pole of the femur, the superior aspect of the joint space, and the acetabulum. As the key weight-bearing components of the hip, these structures are most likely to be involved in AVN, which follows a functional, rather than vascular, anatomic distribution. The addition of coronal and sagittal reconstructions ensure thorough assessment of these structures. MPR best allows appreciation of the true status of the superior pole, joint space, acetabulum, and weight-bearing surface. When early abnormalities involve the superior pole (and in AVN this is usually the case), MPR may confirm or detect abnormalities not well seen on the transaxial images.

Preoperative planning is facilitated by the anatomic analysis provided by CT/MPR. Core decompressions are appropriate and apparently most successful only in those patients with early (CT stage I, IIa, some IIb) AVN, prior to extensive architectural alteration of the head and superior pole. By the time stage IIb or IIIa disease is seen, core decompression may offer symptomatic relief, but many orthopedic surgeons would perform osteotomy as a more definitive procedure. The purpose of an osteotomy is to reposition a more

TABLE 10-1. Revised radiographic staging of AVN, based on CT/MPR criteria

Plain Film Staging	CT/MPR Staging	
	Stage	Definition or Explanation
0 (normal)	0	No change
I (preradiographic)	I	May be defined by future research into density measurement, trabecular assessment, and other factors.
II	IIa	Subtle, early sclerosis and osteoporosis. Trabecular coarsening (altered asterisk sign).
	IIb	Distinct/definite foci of sclerosis, osteoporosis. Early subchondral rim or crescent sign.
III	IIIa	Contour at risk. Advanced subchondral undermining. Large cysts.
	IIIb	Early alterations in contour or subchondral fracture.
IV	IV	Marked collapse of femoral head. Significant acetabular involvement.

Magid D, Fishman EK, Scott WW, et al: Femoral head avascular necrosis: CT assessment with multiplanar reconstruction. Radiology 7(3):741, 1985.

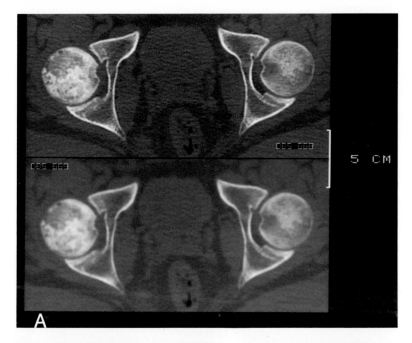

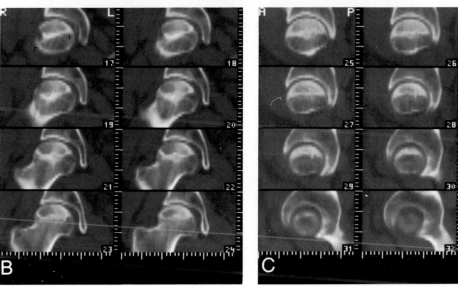

FIG. 10-2. (A) Transaxial CT obtained with high resolution technique (7 sec, 780 mAs, 2 mm collimation) in a 23-year-old man with a history of right hip pain. Bony details are enhanced by high-resolution filter (top two images). There are extensive sclerotic and cystic alterations in the right femoral head compatible with AVN. However, the asymptomatic left hip also shows subtle patchy sclerotic alterations with irregularity of the trabecular "asterisk" pattern. Eight sequential coronal (B) and eight sagittal (C) images map the area of involvement of the right hip and confirm the integrity of the contour and joint space. It would be difficult to find enough normal femoral head to create a new weight-bearing surface. The right hip is stage IIIa, the left is stage IIa.

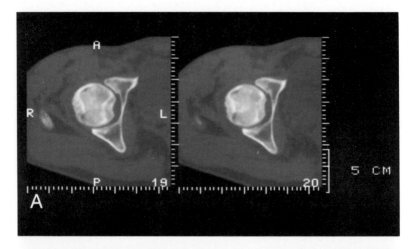

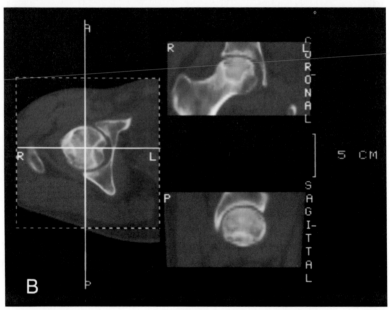

FIG. 10-3. In a 28-year-old man with right hip pain and surgically confirmed AVN, plain films had shown a well-marginated lesion of the femoral head. (A) Two transaxial images through the midfemoral head show extensive geographic lesion with sclerotic margins, involving most of the head at this level. A subtle radiolucent subchondral "crescent sign" is seen anteriorly. (B) Reference transaxial (left) image showing axes from which one coronal (top right) and one sagittal (bottom right) image have been drawn for display. These confirm the extent of this lesion and that the contour and joint space are intact. The coronal view best demonstrates the conical area of involvement and sclerotic margins. This is stage IIIa: extensive involvement with preserved, but threatened, contour.

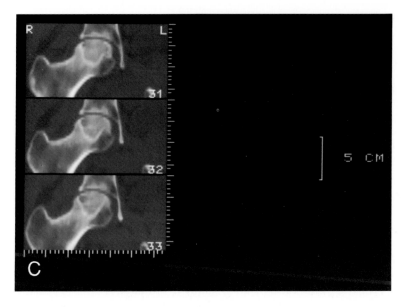

FIG. 10-3. (*continued*).   (C) Three sequential coronal views again demonstrate the matrix, margin, and area of involvement, and confirm preserved joint space, contour, and acetabulum.

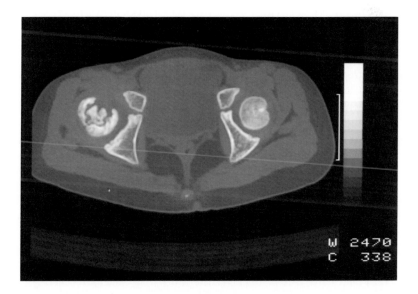

FIG. 10-4.   In a 9-year-old girl with Legg-Calve-Perthes disease, transaxial CT demonstrates collapse of right femoral head with defect in anterior position of femoral head (arrow). Slight deformity of posterior portion of acetabulum is also noted.

normal portion of femoral head in the weight-bearing position. CT/MPR provides a precise anatomic "road map" of femoral head abnormalities, allowing more specific preoperative planning. CT also alters management and operative planning, by revealing more extensive disease than that anticipated from plain films. In some cases, CT/MPR documentation of unanticipated IIb or IIIa disease may lead to osteotomy where core decompression was initially favored, while the discovery of a diffusely abnormal head even with only limited contour alteration (stage IIIb) may lead to arthroplasty rather than previously planned osteotomy. Postoperative CT/MPR may be used to confirm surgical results and to follow the progress of disease. In some cases, we have documented surgical results less satisfactory than anticipated (no real change in the post-osteotomy position of the weight-bearing surface; rapid progression of disease), which allows the surgeon to generate a more conservative but more realistic plan and prognosis.

These patients are at risk for bilateral, often asynchronous, disease. In our first 60 cases of AVN we discovered 9 asymptomatic but abnormal contralateral hips, usually with early disease (stage IIa or IIb). This suggested the possibility of femoral head preservation with prompt treatment.

In reviewing our experience with 60 patients with AVN, we found that CT upgraded staging in one-third of the patients evaluated and, more significantly, altered management plans for 41 percent of the patients evaluated. The discovery of early and asymptomatic disease suggested the potential of CT/MPR to reduce the morbidity of AVN. Finally, with more accurate definition and staging, it may be possible to provide a more meaningful assessment of the efficacies of various currently controversial treatment modalities.

Metallic Hip Implants

One of the surprising results of our evaluation of the MPR/D reconstruction program is its use in the patient with orthopedic hardware. Routine transaxial images through metallic hip implants or prostheses cause significant artifact due to the high CT attenuation of the metal. In many institutions these patients will not be scanned due to the poor image quality of the resultant scans.

Yet by using the MPR/D program the metal-generated artifacts can be significantly reduced. The problem with CT scanning of orthopedic hardware lies in the severe radiographic attenuation (missing data) caused by the metal in certain views. The missing data (hollow projections) create starburst artifacts in the standard axial images. Left uncorrected, these artifacts make it nearly impossible to obtain useful information in the vicinity of the metal implants.

These "starburst" artifacts can be reduced by reformation of the axial CT image data into orthogonal or oblique planes. Data reformation into other planes will weight the true signal over the randomly distributed artifact when one is integrating two adjacent axial images. In this way, the artifact seen in transaxial images is averaged out of the multiplanar reformations. The MPR/D program does this data reformation automatically.[11]

We previously reported our experience with the CT/MPR images in 30 patients with orthopedic hip implants. The metallic devices included total hip replacements (n = 6), one or more surgical plates with screws (n = 9), acetabular pins or screws (n = 9), and Knowles pins (n = 6). In 12 cases the transaxial CT and MPR images received equal grades. However, in 18 of the 30 patients (60 percent), the MPR scored higher. The success of MPR imaging of metallic implants has allowed us to evaluate almost routinely the patient following open reduction with internal fixation of hip fractures (Fig. 10-5, 10-6).

Although the MPR/D program allows reconstructions in any axial or oblique plane, it is still limited by its inability to visualize areas of interest in a dynamic fashion (Figure 10-7). Additionally, although the images present transaxial data in coronal, sagittal, and oblique views, the images are still two-dimensional data presentations. To supplement the MPR/D program, CT manufacturers have developed basic three-dimensional (3D) imaging programs. The two most widely available programs are the Siemens 3D-CT program, developed with Michael Vannier of the Mallincrodt Institute of Radiology,[12,13] and the General Electric 3D83 and 3D98 programs, developed by Gabor Herman and his associates at the University of Pennsylvania.[14-16]

The conventional 3D imaging programs supplied as optimal software on CT scanners by the major vendors (including Siemens Medical Systems and General Electric) rely on thresholding specific levels to highlight the details of the musculoskeletal system. Specific thresholding for bone and soft tissue are chosen in advance and these programs apply sliding algorithms to provide a 3D perspective and a sense of depth.

The Siemans 3D CT is based on level sectioning contour extraction coupled to a nonlinear, noninterpolating asymmetrical digital filter for antialiasing. Density threshold levels that identify bone and soft tissue contours are applied to form three-dimensional images. A nonlinear digital filter is applied to each reconstructed three-dimensional surface image through antialiasing of artifact at the vertical and oblique edges. Surfaces far away from the viewer or reference point appear darker while surfaces that are close appear lighter. An example of such a case is seen in Figure 10-8 in a patient with an acetabular fracture.

In a series of 20 patients by Burke et al.,[17] using standard transaxial images and the GE 3D83 program, all patients with displaced acetabular fractures had the fractures demonstrated by CT scanning. However, in the patients with nondisplaced fractures the fracture lines were poorly demonstrated or, in fact, confused with normal 3D contour lines; in these cases, fracture displacement was usually less than 2 mm. Another limitation of this 3D technique is that the joint space of the hip is obscured by overlapping structures of the 3D image. Although overlapping structures can be removed, the femoral head and its relationship to the joint space were better demonstrated on the routine axial views than on the 3D images.

Since the 3D imaging does not present any new diagnostic information to the radiologist, being only a reformation of the transaxial images, the question often arises as to its clinical utility. In our experience, the primary use has been to further understanding of the pathoanatomy of fractures and complex skeletal structures. This is particularly helpful to practitioners other than radiol-

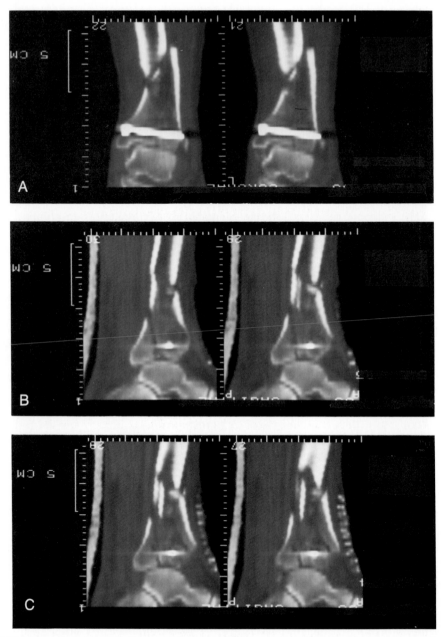

FIG. 10-5. In a 47-year-old man with trimalleolar fracture who had surgery at another hospital, plain films in cast suggested that posterior malleolar fracture had not been reduced. CT scan was done in cast. (A) Coronal scans show satisfactory reduction of medial malleolar fragment. Spiral tibial fracture is clearly seen. Notice only minimal artifact due to metal pin. (B,C) Sagittal views clearly define posterior malleolar fracture (arrows) that has not been stabilized. Sagittal views show full extent of tibial fracture (T, talus). Metal pin does not cause significant artifact.

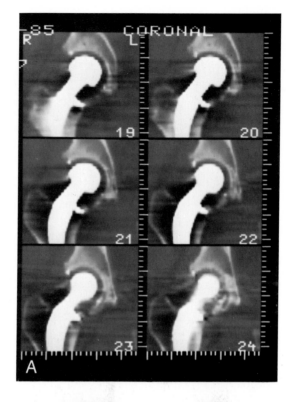

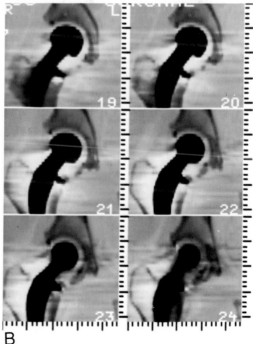

FIG. 10-6. Study of a 54-year-old man with right total hip replacement to evaluate left hip pain. (A) Coronal images show good definition to prosthesis with only minimal loss of data adjacent to metal. (B) Negative mode display of image appears to allow for better definition of edges around prosthesis.

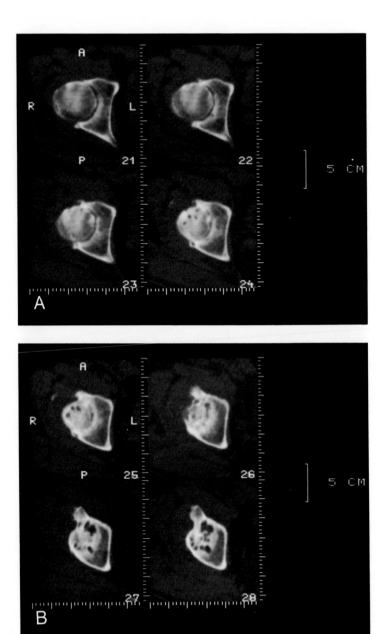

FIG. 10-7. CT scan of a 63-year-old man with osteoarthritis was done to determine the type of surgery needed. Based on coronal and sagittal images, a total hip replacement with acetabular component was chosen. (A,B) Transaxial images demonstrate cystic changes in femoral head and in acetabulum. Extent of joint space narrowing is difficult to determine.

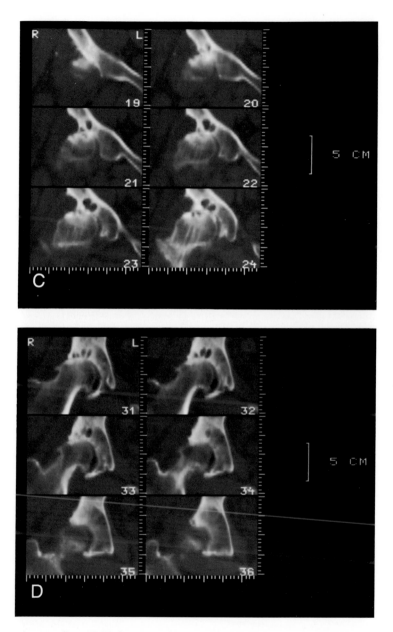

FIG. 10-7. (*continued*).   (C,D) Sequential coronal and sagittal images show cystic changes involving both femoral head and acetabulum. Weight-bearing surface of acetabulum is now laterally placed.

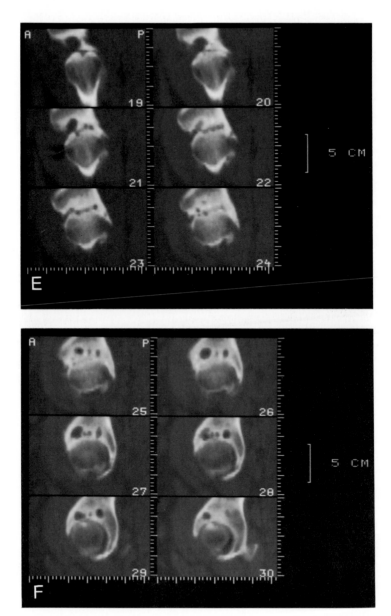

FIG 10-7. (*continued*).   (E,F) Sagittal images are best at defining obliteration of joint space, particularly the anterior portion (arrow).

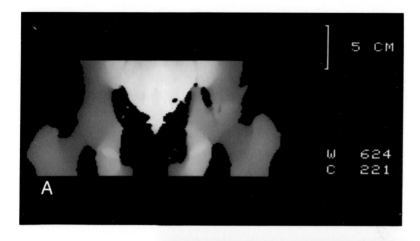

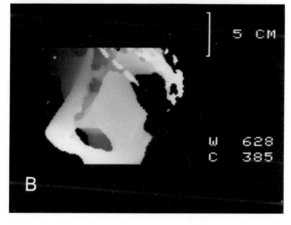

FIG. 10-8. Simulated 3D images produced on Somatom DR-3 scanner of a 45-year-old man with acetabular fracture. Posterior (A) and internal (B) views demonstrate acetabular fracture (arrows). Notice that this technique tends to diminish fine bony details.

ogists who are often at a loss when interpreting the two-dimensional transaxial images and have trouble integrating the information from a series of sequential scans.

Although these images can be helpful, they are still limited by the operator's inability to choose a specific angle or degree of rotation. This problem has been addressed by several manufacturers and has led to the development of free-standing 3D imaging centers. Two leading companies in this field are Cemax Medical Systems (Mountain View, CA) and Dimensional Medicine Systems (Minneapolis, MN).

Image processing on the Cemax 1000 consists of a multiuser 32-bit microprocessor, a 1024 × 1280 display system, and menu-driven software. CT scan data are transferred via magnetic tape. The tape-encoded images from any of the major CT scanners can be interpreted by the system. Each voxel is deconvolved into a symmetrical cube by a linear interpolation scheme and three-dimensional filter. The surface of the desired structure is the isodensity contour that best separates the structure from the surrounding tissues. Ideally, the voxel with a value equal to the half-maximum point of the edge gradient should be selected. The surface contour is computed for each interpolated slice, stacked according to the separation between interpolated slices, and stored as a contour site.

The generation of 3D images is performed from the contour files at any desired projection view (0° to 180°). The images can be displayed under different formats including range encoding, depth-encoded displays, reflectance model, and ring stacking. The number of generalized 3D images is unlimited although time constraints tend to restrict the number of images produced. In our initial experience, the generation of eight images at consecutive 45° of rotation appears satisfactory, although this will obviously vary with other types of pathologic conditions and the requirements of the individual orthopedic surgeon. The images can be viewed on the Cemax 1000 console or on color poloroid film (images in this chapter reproduced in black and white due to publication guidelines). The images are viewed as individual scans; real-time image display is not available.

One valuable feature of the Cemax 1000 system is its ability to remove part of a structure from the whole image. For example, the acetabulum can be viewed directly following removal of the femoral head (Fig. 10-9). Unfortunately, the process is tedious and may take anywhere from 45 to 90 minutes to perform. Further technical improvements to reduce this time interval are being developed.

As with other 3D systems, nondisplaced fractures cannot be detected. In order to detect a fracture there must be a displacement of bone at least 1 pixel wide, because the system uses a surface rendering technique. A volumetric rendering technique would be ideal for use in 3D imaging systems. A volumetric rendering technique that can be used to create three-dimensional views of the musculoskeletal system was developed by the Computer Graphics group at Lucasfilm, Ltd., in 1985.

Volumetric rendering differs from surface rendering in that all of the information from the CT scans can be preserved, not just the surface boundaries, so that object thickness can be seen in the three-dimensional projections. Surface rendering techniques also require boundary detection algorithms to define surfaces. These algorithms work adequately for defining the surfaces of major objects; however, they do not preserve subtle surface detail well, such as bone fractures, which may be less than 1 pixel wide in the CT scans.

In volumetric rendering, the CT scans are conceptually stacked up as a volume in the computer and the grey-scale intensity information of the pixels in the volume is replaced with gels of varying color and transparency. Color views of the volume can be computed from arbitrary three-dimensional angles and with arbitrary degrees of object transparency.

A color and transparency value is chosen for each tissue type in the CT study. Color and transparency values for tissues are chosen based on what we want to accentuate. For example, if we were interested in the relationship

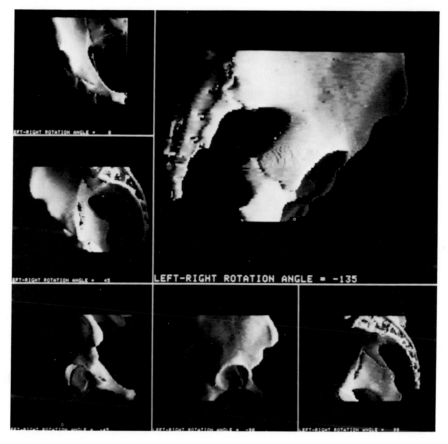

FIG. 10-9. Composite 3D images generated on a Cemax 1000 in a patient with acetabular fracture. On this series of images the femoral head has been removed to allow better definition of the fracture line extending through the acetabulum (arrows).

between muscles and bones, we might choose a semitransparent red to represent muscle, and opaque white to represent bone, and a completely transparent color to represent all other tissues.

Each monochromatic pixel in the volume is replaced by a colored gel pixel. The color and transparency of the gel chosen to replace each pixel are based on the percentages of each tissue type found in the pixel. The percentage of each tissue type present in a pixel is determined by looking at the imaging characteristics of the different tissue types and the intensities of the neighboring pixels. For example, if we decided to represent fat as a very transparent green and soft tissue as an opaque red, and we find that a pixel is 77 percent fat and 23 percent soft tissue, the pixel would be replaced with a translucent yellow gel.

To construct a three-dimensional projection from a given angle, viewing rays are traced from the viewing plane through the colored gel volume. The gels of the tissue types encountered by each ray absorb a certain percentage of the ray, and allow the rest of it to pass through to the next tissue. The more opaque a tissue is, the less can be seen of what is behind it. A conceptual light source can also be defined to shade the volume. Shading can show texture between surfaces in the volume and provide monocular depth cues.

The volumetric rendering technique has been implemented on the Pixar Image Computer, a machine designed for image computing that operates at speeds 200 times the speed of a minicomputer. Typically, a rotation sequence for a volume is computed and then the image computer allows the radiologist or orthopedic surgeon to view the pathologic area interactively as it rotates (Fig. 10-10). The system is presently undergoing clinical trials and we hope that it will be available for widespread clinical use within the next 2 years.

Preoperative Evaluation: Optimal Press–Fit Design

One of the newer uses for CT data has been in designing custom orthopedic implants. One of the problems with standard stock prostheses is that there is a potential for poor fit, resulting in subsequent prosthesis loosening, patient discomfort, or premature metal fatigue. In theory, a custom prosthesis designed to match individual anatomy should be associated with better results.

There is some clinical evidence that the long-term success of noncemented hip stems improves with maximal filling of the femoral canal, and resistance to axial torques. The rationale is that the maximum area of contact on the internal bone surface produces tolerable levels of stress, reduces bone resorption and sinkage, and restricts micromotion that can lead to pain. These design considerations have been incorporated in the newer, more anatomically shaped hip stem designs. While such designs do improve canal fit they still do not provide an exact fit for individual bones. Custom designed implants represent an attempt to do this. However, in the past, custom implants have fallen short of this goal because they used two radiographic images (anteroposterior and lateral) to model the 3D geometry of the bone. Extrapolation from such limited data precludes precise stem–canal fit.[18,19] CT has now allowed us to generate more accurate 3D skeletal models.[18-20] While such information potentially can improve the fit of custom implants, it does not necessarily guarantee optimal fit. The problem is that the three-dimensional curvatures of the canal would require areas of an exactly canal-shaped stem to be removed in order to make insertion possible. Optimal-fit design, the result of combining accurate 3D geometry with optimal mechanics, requires artificial intelligence computer methods to perform the thousands of design choices necessary to achieve the required fit.

Software has been developed at the Orthopedic Biomechanics Laboratory, Brigham and Women's Hospital, to design an optimal-fit custom hip stem based on bone geometry data obtained from CT. Appropriate image processing and contouring algorithms are used to obtain accurate outer femoral shell and

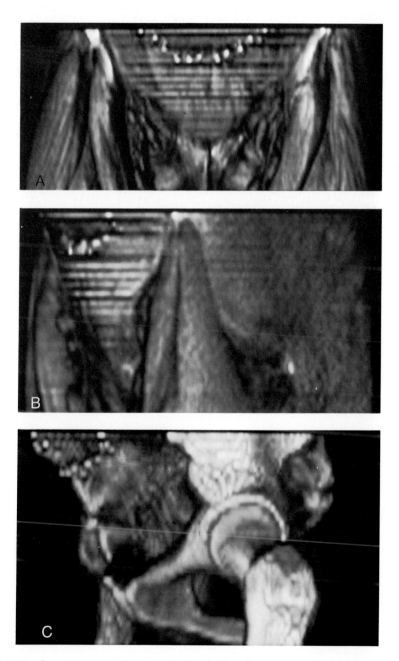

FIG. 10-10. In a 40-year-old woman who had undergone renal transplant surgical clips are noted in midline on 3D image reconstruction done on Pixar (original images are in color). (A) Anterior view clearly defines the major muscle groups of pelvis. (B,C) On the oblique view with soft tissue and bone settings the Pixar allows excellent definition of all tissues, depending on parameter selection.

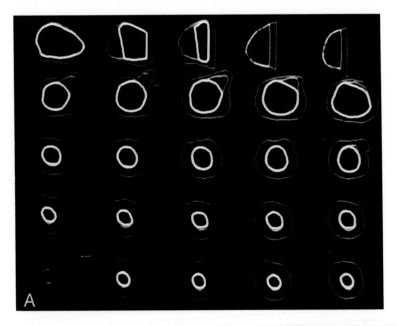

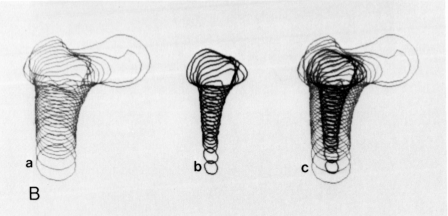

FIG. 10-11. Sequential steps in computer-generated design of custom hip implant. (A) Axial contours of outer cortex, medullary canal, and optimal-fit implants (thick white contours). (B) Bony contours generated from CT scans. (a) Outer cortex; (b) medullary canal; (c) cortex and canal.

inner femoral canal models from the relatively bony dimensions produced from the single-energy CT images.[21] The models consist of multiple axial contours defined by consecutive contour points. Over 1000 polygons are used to describe each model's surface. Computer simulation can then be used to perform trial surgical manipulations of the femur prior to implant insertion. Femoral neck cuts, greater trochanter resection, canal reaming and rasping can all be performed by removing the involved surface polygons. Upon completion of this

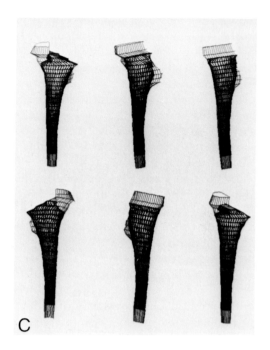

C

FIG. 10-11. (*continued*). (C) Six different views of the canal implant as it rotates towards the viewer. (D) Surface model representation of the computer-designed optimal-fit femoral implant.

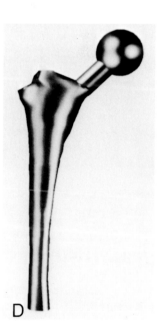

D

simulation module, an optimal press-fit implant can be designed integrating geometric, mechanical, and surgical demands (Fig. 10-11).

Some stem areas must be removed to allow insertion. Therefore it is important to identify and retain those stem areas that optimize stem–bone load transfer conditions and minimize stem motion. Optimal load transfer to axial forces and bending moments is achieved by maintaining exact fit along the proximal medial wall and calcar of the femur. A further requirement is to ensure that the stem does not wedge distally within the canal. To prevent medial–lateral rocking, contact at the distal lateral tip of the stem is maintained. Stem filling of the proximal canal is also a high priority because it helps to achieve axial torsional stability for the stem and axial load-bearing in that region. Various areas of the canal surface model are then scored, with higher scores being assigned to critical areas as described above. These higher scores will ensure preservation of ideal fit at critical points as the stem is modified and reduced to allow surgical insertion.

The design process begins with an ideal initial stem model, that is, one completely filling the canal. The modification process begins with translation of the stem an incremental amount up the vertical axis of the canal. The stem is then moved in small increments in each of the other five degrees of freedom (three rotations and two translations). At each given orientation where the stem intersects or impinges on the canal surface, a canal–stem surface overlap score is determined. This score is calculated by summing all the polygons that overlap at each point, weighted by the priority score. Highly scored points would produce a high overlap score when shaved off; stem reduction obtained by minimization of score ensures preservation of important stem areas. The movement that produced the minimum overlap score is flagged and the stem is moved to this position. All areas of overlap are then shaved away and the stem model is once again completely within the canal. This process is repeated until the entire stem has passed through the proximal femoral neck cut. The resultant stem shape describes the optimal canal–stem fit that comes closest to the biomechanical ideal while still being insertable through the proximal femur.

Once generated, the bone and stem model data are used as input for computer graphics modeling and finite element analysis. Computer graphic methods are used for visualization and for qualitative assessments of stem–bone fit. Finite element analysis is used to examine the mechanical environment of the stem and bone. The data are also entered into a numerically controlled milling machine, which produces an actual bone model and optimal-fit hip stem for surgical implantation. This work has also been applied to the design of total knee replacements.

CONCLUSIONS

The radiologic evaluation of musculoskeletal disorders is undergoing a rapid metamorphosis due to the development of new imaging modalities such as CT and magnetic resonance imaging, as well as computer-driven programs for advanced data manipulation.[22] We must not forget that the object of these technical advances is better radiologic diagnostic and presurgical planning capabilities, resulting in better patient care. As we illustrate in this chapter, this undoubtedly is the case.

REFERENCES

1. Glenn WV, Rhodes ML, Altschuler EM et al: Multiplanar display computerized body tomography applications in the lumbar spine. Spine 4:(4)282, 1979

2. Glenn VW, Rhodes ML, Rothman SLG: The ultimate CT image. p. 25 In Littleton JT, Durizch JL (eds): Sectional Imaging Methods. University Park Press, Baltimore, 1983

3. Magid D, Fishman EK, Scott WW, Jr., et al: Femoral heal avascular necrosis: CT assessment with multiplanar reconstruction. Radiology 157:751, 1985

4. Fishman EK, Magid D, Mandelbaum BR: RadioGraphics 6:7, 1986

5. Hungerford DS: Treatment of ischemic necrosis of the femoral head. p. 5 In Evarts CM (ed): Surgery of the Musculoskeletal System. Churchill Livingstone, New York, 1983

6. D'Aubigne RM, Postel M, Mazabraud A, et al: Idiopathic necrosis of the femoral head in adults. J Bone Joint Surg 47B(4):612, 1965

7. Steinberg ME, Brighton CT, Steinberg DR et al: Treatment of avascular necrosis of the femoral head by a combination of bone grafting, decompression and electrical stimulation. Clin Orthop Rel Res 186:137, 1984

8. Conklin JJ, Alderson PO, Zizic TM et al: Comparison of bone scan and radiographic sensitivity in the detection of steroid-induced ischemic necrosis of bone. Radiology 147:221, 1983

9. Dihlmann W: CT analysis of the upper end of the femur: the asterisk sign and ischemic necrosis of the femoral head. Skel Radiol 8:251, 1982

10. Resnik CS, Resnik D, Pineda C et al: Femoral trabecular analysis by computed tomography. Exhibit presented at the 70th Scientific Assembly & Annual Meeting of the Radiological Society of North America, Washington, DC November 1984

11. Fishman EK, Magid D, Robertson DD et al: CT/MPR imaging of metallic hip implants. Radiology Sept 1986 (In press).

12. Totty WG, Vannier MW: Complex musculoskeletal anatomy: analysis using three dimensional surface reconstructions. Radiology 150:173, 1984

13. Vannier MW, Marsh JL, Warren JO: Three-dimensional CT reconstruction images for craniofacial surgical planning and evaluation. Radiology 150:179, 1984

14. Chen LS, Herman GT, Meyer CR, Udupa JK: 3D 98—an easy to use software package for three dimensional display from computed tomograms. Proc SPIE 515:309, 1984

15. Chen LS, Herman GT, Meyer CR, Udupa JK: 3D 98—an easy to use software package for three dimensional display of organs on the GE 9800 CT scanner. Radiology 153:183, 1985

16. Herman GT, Liv HK: Display of three dimensional information in computed tomography. J Comput Assist Tomogr 1: 155, 1977

17. Burk DL, Jr., Mears DC, Kennedy WH et al: Three dimensional computed tomography of acetabular fractures. Radiology 155:183, 1985

18. Nerubay J, Robinstein Z, Katznelson A: Technique of building a hemipelvic prosthesis using computed tomography. Prog Clin Biol Res 99:147, 1981

19. Woolson S, Dev P, Fellingham L, Vassiliadis A: Three-dimensional imaging of bone from computerized tomography. Clin Orthop Rel Res 202:239, 1986

20. Rhodes ML, Azzawi Y, Chu E, et al: Anatomic model and prosthesis manufacturing using CT data. Proc Nat Computer Graphics Assoc 3:110, 1985

21. Robertson DD, Huang HK: Quantitative measurement of bone using CT with second order correction. Med Phys (In press).

22. D'Agincourt LG, Hess TP: 3D and multiplanar CT market: a puzzle for manufacturers. Diag Imaging 7(7):46, 1985

CASE NO. 1 Charles Diana

History of Renal Failure with Bone Pain and Vomiting in a 33-Year-Old Man

A 33-year-old black man with a 20-year history of renal failure had been on dialysis for 4 years. Complaints of chronic bone pain, tremors, nausea, and vomiting, coupled with elevated serum calcium and phosphate levels, led to the diagnosis of secondary hyperparathyroidism. Surgery produced 927 mg hyperplastic parathyroid tissue (normal, 120 to 130 mg). A scan of the pelvis was obtained due to increasing left hip pain (Figs. 1 and 2).

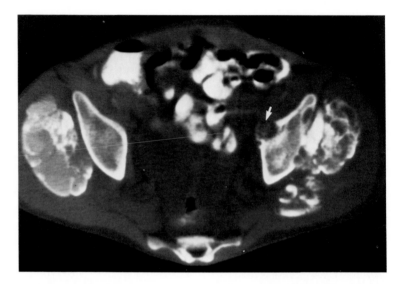

FIGURE 1   Transaxial image through the acetabular roof, viewed at bone windows. There are large, lobular, heterogenous radiodensities lateral to both ilia compatible with periarticular soft tissue calcifications. These have an indolent appearance, with denser rim calcifications and no evidence of invasion or infiltration—as opposed to bulk displacement—of adjacent muscle masses. The left ilium shows scalloped cortical erosion posterolaterally, possibly by this mass, and there are low-density lytic lesions of the anterolateral and anteromedial (arrow) margins.

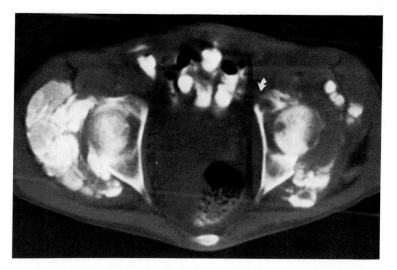

FIGURE 2   Transaxial image through the midacetabulum again shows the extensive, lobular periarticular soft tissue calcifications and demonstrates another lytic and minimally expansile lesion of the left anterior column (arrow).

DISCUSSION

The CT scan shows extensive calcification of soft tissues around both hip joints. There are several lytic lesions of the left acetabulum, consistent with brown tumor. While the differential diagnosis of periarticular soft tissue calcifications is large, the presence of these lytic lesions narrows the differential diagnosis considerably, making renal osteodystrophy with secondary or tertiary hyperparathyroidism the most likely diagnosis.

Renal osteodystrophy is used to describe the bone disease characteristic of patients with chronic renal failure. It is a complex disease, resulting from a combination of biochemical abnormalities.

Radiologic Findings in Renal Osteodystrophy

Rickets and Osteomalacia

Found in children and adults respectively, these conditions are characterized by poor mineralization of bone osteoid. In general, the changes seen with rickets and osteomalacia are seen in disease states characterized by low levels of serum calcium and/or phosphorus. They may or may not be associated with low levels of vitamin D. The cause of rickets and osteomalacia are often divided into vitamin D-dependent and vitamin D-resistant groups.

Patients with renal failure develop decreased levels of vitamin D and calcium by three interrelated means: (1) Since the calcium phosphorus (CaxP) product is maintained below 60 to 70 (the level at which precipitation occurs), hyperphosphatemia secondary to decreased renal excretion directly lowers serum calcium; (2) hyperphosphatemia inhibits vitamin D activation, slowing intestinal absorption of calcium, and (3) direct renal activation of vitamin D decreases with declining renal function.

In renal osteodystrophy, radiologic findings due to rickets are most apparent in areas of rapid growth, such as the knee joint, and include widened growth plate, irregular zone of provisional calcification (distal metaphysis), and metaphyseal cupping and fraying. Bowing of long bones and diffuse bony demineralization are common. Slipped capital femoral epiphysis may occur.

The changes in adults due to osteomalacia include osteopenia and pseudofractures, or Looser's zones. There are linear horizontal radiolucencies across bones that represent focal areas of unmineralized osteoid. They occur most commonly in the medial scapula, ribs, and pubic and ischial rami.

Secondary Hyperparathyroidism

Patients in renal failure are often hypocalcemic. This hypocalcemia stimulates the parathyroid glands to produce excess parathyroid hormone, resulting in secondary hyperparathyroidism. Although it is most commonly seen in renal failure, other hypocalcemic syndromes such as malabsorption may cause hyperparathyroidism. If hyperparathyroidism persists despite correction of serum calcium levels, the condition is called tertiary hyperparathyroidism.

Several radiologic changes in renal osteodystrophy can be attributed to secondary hyperparathyroidism, including

1. Subperiosteal bone resorption, most commonly along the radial aspect of the phalanges of the hand. It may also occur at the distal end of the clavicles, medial tibia, medial humerus, and distal ulna. Resorption of distal phalangeal tufts may be seen.
2. Subchondral and subligamentous bone resorption, characterized by widening of the symphysis pubis and sacroiliac joints, and bony resorption on the ischial tuberosities.
3. Granular "salt and pepper" skull.
4. Generalized osteopenia.
5. Loss of lamina dura on dental radiographs.
6. Brown tumors (expansile lytic lesions) can be seen in any bone.
7. Chondrocalcinosis.

The last two are more common in primary hyperparathyroidism.

Osteosclerosis

One of the most common radiologic findings in patients with renal osteodystrophy is increased bony density, particularly in the vertebral bodies, pelvis, and femurs. This is the cause of the well-known "rugger-jersey spine."

Soft Tissue and Vascular Calcification

Soft tissue calcification in renal failure is both metastatic (due to elevated calcium/phosphorus product) and dystrophic (due to tissue injury) in nature. The major cause is probably hyperphosphatemia with resultant metastatic calcification. It occurs characteristically in five types:

1. Arteries: unlike diabetic calcification, without associated distal ischemia
2. Ocular
3. Periarticular: fluffy, amorphous, "tumoral" calcification
4. Cutaneous and subcutaneous
5. Visceral: amorphous calcinosis

Differential Diagnosis of Soft Tissue Calcifications

Soft tissue calcification can be organized into four general categories.

In soft tissue ossification, true trabeculated bone is formed. Causes include myositis ossificans progressiva and circumscripta, paralysis, soft tissue sarcomas, and parosteal osteosarcoma. Surgical scars may ossify, and heterotopic bone may form in severely burned patients.

Metabolic disease with elevation of the calcium/phosphate product above 60 to 70 produces metastatic calcification of normal tissues. Causes include pseudohypoparathyroidism, hypervitaminosis D, milk-alkali syndrome, renal osteodystrophy with secondary hyperparathyroidism, diffuse bony metastases with hypercalcemia, and sarcoid.

Dystrophic calcification occurs in injured tissues. Causes include tissue infarction, such as in myocardial infarction, calcific tendinitis or bursitis, and necrotic tumors. Connective tissue disorders such as scleroderma, dermatomyositis, and systemic lupusery thematosis may cause soft tissue calcification.

Calcinosis is true idiopathic calcification, without known tissue injury or metabolic disturbance. The best known causes are rare disorders: tumoral calcinosis and calcinosis universals. The connective tissue decreases are sometimes included here.

Final diagnosis: Renal osteodystrophy with secondary hyperparathyroidism.

REFERENCES 1. Bricker NS, Slatopolsky E, Reiss E, Avioli LV: Calcium, phosphorus and bone in renal disease and transplantation. Arch Intern Med 123:543, 1969

2. Mankin H: Rickets, osteomalacia and renal osteodystrophy. J Bone Joint Surg 56A:101, 1974

3. Parfitt AM: Soft tissue calcification in uremia. Arch Intern Med 124:544, 1969

4. Resnick D, Niwayama G. Diagnosis of Bone and Joint Disorders. WB Saunders, Philadelphia, 1981.

5. Siegelman SS: Osteoporosis, osteomalacia, and hyperparathyroidism. p. 153 In Feldman F (ed): Radiology, Immunology and Pathology of Bones and Joints. Appleton-Century-Crofts, New York, 1978

6. Weller M, Edeiken J, Hodes PJ: Renal osteodystrophy. Am J Roentgenol 104(2):354, 1968

CASE NO. 2   Edward Farmlett

Pelvis and Lower Back Pain in a 59-Year-Old Man

A 59-year-old man presented with pain in the pelvis and lower back. The patient had had increasing constipation over the previous 6 months. A CT scan was then done (Fig. 1).

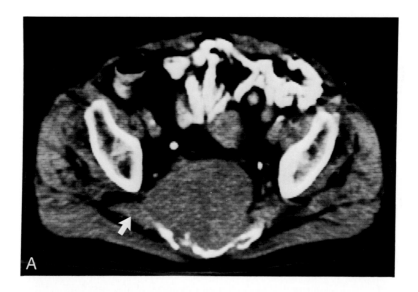

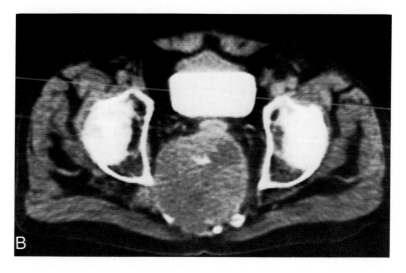

FIGURE 1   (A,B) Large necrotic tumor is seen invading and destroying the sacrum. Tumor extends into the right sacrosciatic foramen (arrow).

DISCUSSION

Chordoma is a rare, locally invasive, indolent malignancy arising from notochord remnants. The notochord makes a brief appearance during the fourth to seventh week of embryonic development, leaving the centrum of the nucleus pulposis as its only structural derivative. However, small rests of notochord occasionally can be found in the adult from the clivis to the coccyx. Chordomas are believed to arise within these rests, or within the nucleus pulposi, since almost all of these tumors occur in the axial skeleton and resemble embryonic notochord histologically.[1-3]

Chordomas account for 3 to 4 percent of primary malignant neoplasms of bone.[3] Chordomas can occur at any age, but occur predominantly in the fifth to seventh decades[1,4,5] and are rare in patients under the age of 30.[3,5] Approximately 50 percent of chordomas occur in the sacrococcygeal region, 35 percent in the clivus, and 15 percent in the remainder of the vertebral column.[3-6] Chordomas occurring in the sacrum are twice as common in men than women,[1,3-6] while intracranial chordomas occur without predilection for sex and at a younger mean age.[1]

Low back pain is the most common symptom of sacrococcygeal chordomas.[5] Constipation is a common early complaint, with fecal incontinence occurring late in the course of the disease.[5,7] Urinary symptoms such as frequency, urgency, and straining on micturation become increasingly prominent with time.[5,7] Sciatica is occasionally seen due to involvement of pelvic nerves.[7] In most cases, digital rectal examination reveals a firm, lobular mass fixed to the sacrum and extrinsic to the rectum.[1,7]

The most common radiographic finding in sacrococcygeal chordoma is lytic bone destruction of several sacral segments with an associated anterolateral soft tissue mass, which can extend superiorly and inferiorly.[3-5,8] Computed tomography is very useful for surgical and radiotherapy planning in the evaluation of the extent of this mass.[9] CT numbers usually range from 20 to 250 HU, and in 50 percent of cases the mass contains one or more areas of low attenuation which help to confirm the diagnosis of chordoma.[8] These low-density areas probably represent the semiliquid or gelatinous material seen on gross pathologic examination of the surgical specimen.[3,5,8] Amorphous calcification may be scattered throughout the tumor, with the reported incidence[3,5,7,8] ranging from 15 to 89 percent. In addition to the primary bone-destructive changes, areas of secondary sclerosis may be seen in approximately half of the cases, especially in the periphery.[1,5] The tumor frequently extends into the sacral canal, especially in recurrent cases, and can involve the posterior spinous elements as well as extending into the soft tissues posterior to the sacrum.[5,8] The soft tissue mass can grow quite large in the pelvis by the time of diagnosis, and frequently displaces the rectum and bladder. Although invasion of the rectum may be extensive, ulceration of the mucosa is very rare.[1] The radiographic differential diagnosis of sacrococcygeal chordoma includes giant cell tumor, plasmacytoma, metastatic adenocarcinoma, chrondrosarcoma, and osteomyelitis.[1,8]

Although chordomas are indolent tumors, their local aggressiveness and high incidence of postoperative recurrence (85 percent) have led to a poor prognosis.[4,5,8] The incidence of distant metastases in the literature ranges from 10[1] to 43 percent,[6] with an average of approximately 30 percent. The metastases are most commonly spread hematogenously to the lung, lymph nodes, bone, liver, and skin.[4,5,7] The 5-year survival for adults with the diagnosis of sacrococcygeal chordoma is 66 percent,[5,9] with an average survival of 7 years.[6] Chordomas are rare in children, but when they occur are highly malignant and rapidly fatal.[10]

Since chordomas are potentially recurrent malignant lesions, and since their postoperative behavior can not be accurately predicted histologically,[4] the treatment of choice traditionally has been wide local resection followed by postoperative radiation.[1,6] This excision is difficult and usually incomplete; thus care by surgery is rare.[5,6] In addition, chordomas are relatively radioresistant, and thus postoperative radiation also is palliative, not curative.[7] However, some reports indicate that early diagnosis combined with radical surgery may be curative.[3,7] Despite the morbidity of such procedures, these radical surgical techniques may improve the otherwise poor prognosis for patients with sacrococcygeal chordomas.

Final diagnosis: Sacrococcygeal chordoma.

REFERENCES   1. Firooznia H, Pinto RS, Lin JP et al: Chordoma: radiologic evaluation of 20 cases. Am J Roentgenol 127:797, 1976

2. Utne JR, Pugh DG: The roentgenologic aspects of chordoma. Am J Roentgenol 74:593, 1955

3. Dahlin DC: Bone Tumors: General Aspects and Data on 6,221 Cases, 3rd ed. Charles C Thomas, Springfield, Ill., 1978

4. Volpe R, Mazabraud A: A clinicopathologic review of 25 cases of chordoma (a pleomorphic and metastasizing neoplasm). Am J Surg Pathol 7(2):161, 1983

5. Sundaresan N, Galich JH, Chu FCH, Huvos AG: Spinal chordomas. J Neurosurg 50:312, 1979

6. Higinbotham NL, Phillips RF, Farr HW, Hustu HO: Chordoma: thirty-five year study at Memorial Hospital. Cancer 20:1841, 1967

7. Mindell ER: Current concepts review: chordoma. J Bone Joint Surg 63 A (3):501, 1981

8. Meyer JE, Lepke RA, Lindfors KK et al: Chordomas: their CT appearance in the cervical, thoracic and lumbar spine. Radiology 153:693, 1984

9. Hudson TM, Galceran M: Radiology of sacrococcygeal chordoma. Clin Ortho Rel Res 175:237, 1983

10. Richards AT, Stricke L, Spitz L: Sacrococcygeal chordomas in children. J Pediatr Surg 8:911, 1973

CASE NO. 3   Alma Lynch-Nyhan

Knee Pain in a 50-Year-Old Man

A 50-year-old white man presented for evaluation of left knee pain of 6-months' duration. Radiographs of the distal left femur showed a destructive lytic bone lesion, and a bone infarction more proximally. CT demonstrated multiple bone infarcts in both femurs, and an aggressive lytic lesion in the distal left femur (Figs. 1, 2). No significant soft tissue mass was associated with this process. The major differential diagnoses included malignant fibrous histiocytoma, osteogenic sarcoma, and chondrosarcoma.

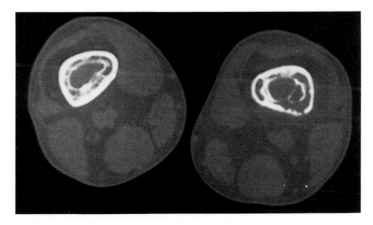

FIGURE 1   Distal femoral diphysis. Both femora show irregular endosteal thickening and sclerosis compatible with bilateral bone infarcts. There is no evidence of periosteal reaction or soft tissue involvement.

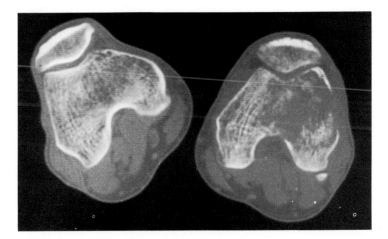

FIGURE 2   Distal femoral condyles. The right side is normal. There is an eccentric lytic lesion predominantly involving the left lateral condyle, which has broken through the cortex laterally and posteromedially. Tissue windows demonstrate only minimal soft tissue swelling and no defninite soft tissue mass or calcifications.

DISCUSSION

Malignant fibrous histiocytoma (MFH) is well known among the tumors of somatic soft tissues, but only recently has it been recognized as a primary tumor of bone. It is a neoplasm of mesenchymal origin. Both the benign and malignant forms are spindle-cell neoplasms in which fascicles of cells exhibit a "storiform" or "cartwheel" arrangement. In addition to fibroblasts and histiocyte-like cells, other cellular components such as myxoid, foam, inflammatory, and giant cells are contained in these tumors.

Up to 1984, only 200 cases of primary malignant fibrous histiocytoma of bone had been reported in the world literature. Of these, only 13 cases are known to have occurred in association with a bone infarction. Malignant fibrous histiocytoma arising in normal bone tends to be evenly distributed between the second and sixth decades. Generally, MFH arising in a pre-existing bone abnormality (i.e., in pagetic bone, previously irradiated bone, dedifferentiated chondrosarcoma, bone infarction, osteochondroma, enchondroma, nonossifying fibroma, chordoma, neurofibromatosis, or bone cyst), occurs in older persons.

The male–female ratio is about equal. As with osteosarcoma and fibrosarcoma, the bones around the knee joint tend to be affected most often (approximately 50 percent of cases).

Radiologically, MFH usually presents as a purely lytic aggressive metaphyseal lesion, often extending into soft tissue. The margins tend to be ill-defined. Periosteal reaction is rare. Pathologic fracture occurs in approximately 20 percent of cases.

Treatment is usually surgical. Adjuvant chemotherapy and/or radiotherapy may be used. An MFH arising in pre-existing bone abnormalities has a worse prognosis than MFH arising in normal bone. In one study the 3-year survival rate was 18 percent for primary MFH arising in abnormal bone versus 43 percent overall 3-year survival rate for all cases studied.

Final diagnosis: Malignant fibrous histiocytoma.

REFERENCES   1. Capanna R, Bertoni F, Bacchini P et al: Malignant fibrous histiocytoma of bone. Cancer 54:177, 1984

2. Nakashima Y, Morishita S, Morishita S et al: Malignant fibrous histiocytoma of bone. Cancer 55:2804, 1985

3. Ros P, Viamonte M, Rywlin A: Malignant fibrous histocytoma: mesenchymal tumor of ubiquitous origin. AJR 142:753, 1984

4. Heselson NG, Price SK, Mills EED et al: Two malignant fibrous histiocytomas in bone infarcts. J Bone Joint Surg 65A: 8:1166, 1983

5. Taconis WK, Mulder JD: Fibrosarcoma and malignant fibrous histiocytoma of long bones: radiographic features and grading. Skeletal Radiol 11:237, 1984

CASE NO. 4   Janet Kuhlman

Persistent Hip Pain without a History of Trauma in a 31-Year-Old Man

A 31-year-old man presented with a 3-month history of persistent, disabling left hip pain. He gave no history of antecedent trauma or systemic illness. Onset of his pain was spontaneous and progressed over a 3-month period, with symptoms aggravated by motion and weight bearing. Due to increasing spasm and weakness, the patient developed a limp and required crutches for ambulation. On physical exam, the patient had no fever or local warmth about the hip to suggest infection, and findings on laboratory examination including a white blood cell count and sedimentation rate were normal.

Initial radiographs of the left hip at the onset of symptoms were interpreted as normal. A radionuclide bone scan obtained 1 month after the onset of symptoms and prior to any plain film findings demonstrated diffusely increased radiotracer uptake in the region of the femoral head, and a diagnosis of "early avascular necrosis" was suggested. Because of the unusual features of the case, a CT scan with MRP imaging was performed for further clarification (Fig. 1).

The CT scan demonstrated a large zone of homogeneous osteoporosis involving much of the femoral head. Although the subchondral bone plate was thinned and ill-defined in some areas, the femoral head contour remained completely intact, without deformity. There were no areas of subchondral bone collapse or undermining characteristic of avascular necrosis. Joint space narrowing and effusion were not seen.

Subsequent plain films taken at monthly intervals eventually showed the development of progressive osteoporosis of the left femoral head.

The patient was treated with analgesics and non-weight-bearing. Over the next 4 months, his symptoms gradually resolved and radiographs of his left hip returned to normal.

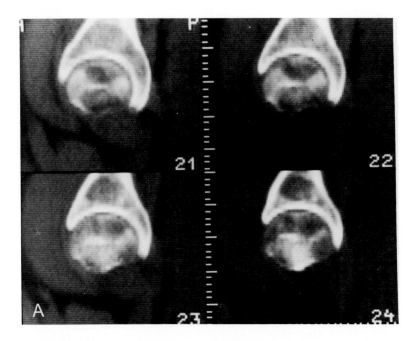

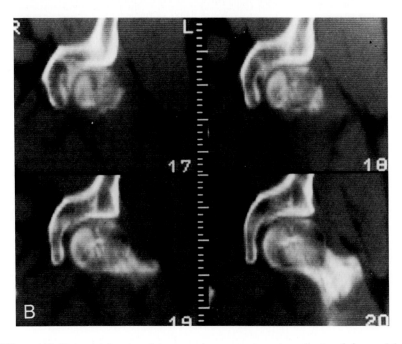

FIGURE 1 (A) Sequential coronal images demonstrate osteoporosis of femoral head and neck region near major weight-bearing surface. (B) Sequential saggital images show extensive osteoporosis of femoral head. No evidence of subcondral collapse is seen.

DISCUSSION

Transient osteoporosis of the hip (TOH) was first described in 1959 by Curtiss and Kincaid in pregnant women during their third trimester.[1] Since then, the majority of reported cases have been in middle-aged men with no history of precipitating trauma or systemic illness.[2-4] Clinical patterns and course of this disease are characteristic, but early symptoms can be confusing and may mimic several other disease processes. Spontaneous onset of hip and groin pain, followed by rapid development of disability, limp, and decreased range of motion are common findings.[2-4] Disability is typically out of proportion to pain, making ambulation difficult. Laboratory examinations are usually normal.[4]

Plain film findings of TOH are rarely evident at the onset of the illness and usually take 3 to 6 weeks to become apparent.[2-5] At that point, radiographs usually show progressive marked osteoporosis of the femoral head with lesser involvement of the adjacent acetabulum and femoral neck. Blurring of the cortical outline of the femoral head without evidence of subchondral bone collapse or deformity is a characteristic finding. Joint space narrowing is notably absent.[2,3,5]

Bone scintigraphy has been reported to be positive early in the course of TOH, prior to plain film changes.[6-8] Positive bone scans show diffusely increased radiotracer uptake involving the entire femoral head, with lesser degrees of abnormal uptake in the acetabulum and femoral shaft.[7] Absence of focal cold spots or inhomogeneity in tracer uptake is reported to be a distinguishing characteristic from early avascular necrosis.[7] However, considerable overlap exists between the scintigraphic findings of AVN and TOH.

In addition to transient osteoporosis of the hip, the differential diagnosis of a painful hip with localized demineralization would initially include several other considerations: septic or tuberculous arthritis, monoarticular rheumatoid arthritis, metastatic involvement, reflex sympathetic dystrophy, disuse atrophy, synovial chondromatosis, villonodular synovitis, and avascular necrosis.[2,3,6] Most of these entities can be differentiated on clinical, laboratory, and radiographic grounds. Septic arthritis would be the most important entity to exclude at first presentation. Absence of fever, systemic symptoms, or elevated white count on sedimentation rate would make an infectious cause less likely, but definitive exclusion of an occult infection would require aspiration of the hip joint for culture.

Perhaps the most difficult differential diagnosis to make is between TOH and early avascular necrosis (AVN).[3,6] Since treatment and prognosis are quite different, the distinction is important. Plain film findings of osteoporosis and lack of joint space narrowing, along with increased radiotracer uptake on bone scans, are common to both TOH and AVN. In difficult cases, CT of the hip with multiplanar reconstruction imaging may be helpful in making the distinction. As illustrated in the present case of TOH, CT demonstrated a pattern of involvement of the femoral head distinctly different from early AVN. Even during the asymptomatic stage of AVN, CT with MPR can detect subtle cystic and sclerotic changes, and early subchondral undermining, better and earlier than plain films.[9] The remarkable feature of this case was the complete preservation of femoral head contour in the presence of marked homogeneous osteoporosis. Because CT scanning is far more sensitive to subtle changes in bone density and bony contour, CT with MPR may be a useful adjuvant to plain films and nuclear scintigraphy in evaluating the painful hip of unknown or elusive cause.

Transient osteoporosis of the hip is a self-limited disease with symptoms lasting 2 to 6 months.[2-4,10] Resolution of radiographic findings lags behind symptom recovery, but is eventually complete without permanent sequelae. Up to 30 percent of patients may go on to develop similar symptoms in the opposite hip.[4] Open biopsy is nondiagnostic and usually not indicated in this self-limited disease.[4] Treatment of TOH consists of supportive measures, with rest and non-weight-bearing recommended to prevent hip fractures, a reported complication.[4,11]

The cause of TOH is unknown. It shares many similarities with regional migratory osteoporosis and may represent the effects of neurovascular compromise, a nontraumatic form of Sudeck's atrophy.[2-6,10,11]

Final diagnosis: Transient osteoporosis of the hip.

REFERENCES   1. Curtiss PH, Kincaid WE: Transitory demineralization of the hip in pregnancy. J Bone Joint Surg 41A:1327, 1959

2. Lequesne M. Transient osteoporosis of the hip: a nontraumatic variety of Sudeck's atrophy. Ann Rheum Dis 27:463, 1968

3. Resnick D, Niwayama G: Diagnosis of Bone and Joint Disorders. WB Saunders, Philadelphia, 1981

4. Kaplan SS, Stegman CJ: Transient osteoporosis of the hip. J Bone Joint Surg 67(3):490, 1985

5. Rosen RA: Transitory demineralization of the femoral head. Radiology 94:509, 1970

6. Bray ST, Partain CL, Teates CD et al: The value of the bone scan in idiopathic regional migratory osteoporosis. J Nucl Med 20:1268, 1979

7. Gaucher A, Colomb J, Naon A et al: The diagnostic value of 99m Tc- diphosophonate bone imaging in transient osteoporosis of the hip. J Rheumatol 6:574, 1979

8. Tannebaum H, Esdaile J, Rosenthall L: Joint imaging in regional migratory osteoporosis. J Rheumatol 7(2):37, 1980

9. Magid D, Fishman EK, Scott WW et al: Femoral head avascular necrosis CT assessment with multiplanar reconstruction. Radiology 157:751, 1985

10. Pantazopoulous T, Exorchou E, Hartofilakidis-Garofalidis G: Idiopathic transient osteoporosis of the hip. J Bone Joint Surg 55A:315, 1973

11. Karasick D, Edeiken J: Case Report 19. Skeletal Radiol 1:181, 1977

CASE NO. 5   Faith Farley

Osteogenic Sarcoma Arising in Irradiated Bone in a 52-Year-Old Woman

A 52-year-old woman had stage IC cervical cancer diagnosed in 1961. She received 4,650 rads external beam radiation and 2 doses of 30 mg intracavitary and 40 mg contracervical radium implants. In March 1984 she presented with sharp pain in her left hip.

A CT scan of the pelvis (Fig. 1) demonstrated a lytic lesion in the left iliac bone involving the acetabular roof (arrows). CT scans through the femoral heads showed increased sclerosis in the left femoral head and neck.

At surgery, the patient was found to have an osteogenic sarcoma of the ischium extending to the pubic ramus and iliac crest with focal vascular and soft tissue invasion and involvement of the gluteus medius and minimus muscles. There were also changes of the femoral head and shaft compatible with Paget's disease.

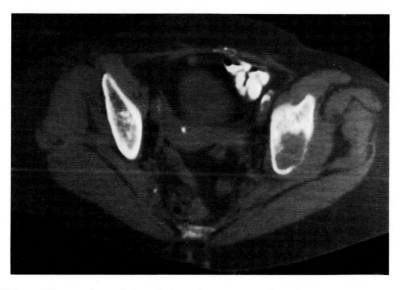

FIGURE 1   CT scan through acetabulum demonstrates lytic lesion in left acetabulum with soft tissue mass.

DISCUSSION

Advances in oncology and radiation therapy have led to increased survival in many forms of cancer, but are also responsible for unfavorable side effects. Recognized complications in adults include radiation necrosis and radiation-induced neoplasms.

Radiation osteitis is a term first used by Ewing to describe the dose-related effects of radiation on bone.[1] Included in the osseous abnormalities are temporary growth cessation with recovery, periostitis, increased fragility with sclerosis, aseptic necrosis, and osteoradionecrosis. Ewing believed that the radiation led to vascular compromise with obliterative endarteritis and periarteritis, which predisposed the patient to infection and osteoradionecrosis.[1] A further complication of the radiation-induced vascular changes is secondary damage to osteoblasts, leading to decreased matrix production.[2-4] Sengupta and Prathap report three cases with no viable osteoblasts in the presence of normal blood vessels.[5]

Radiation effects on bone are dependent on dose and quality of radiation.[4] Excessive total radiation dose, repeated treatment courses, overlapping fields, and orthovoltage treatment appear to be major contributors to radiation osteitis.[4] Cellular damage is most pronouced when dosage exceeds 1,200 rads; the potential for histologic recovery is retained at 600 to 1,200 rads.[6] With supervoltage therapy, smaller therapy fields can be used to achieve desired tumor dose, thereby causing less damage to surrounding structures.[6] Radiation changes have been found to decrease when a given dose is protracted.[6] Radiation effects on growing bone are more profound in periosteal bone formation than enchondral bone growth.[2,7] Young children are most severely affected, although severe changes are also common with irradiation at the time of the adolescent growth spurt.[6,7]

Radiation-induced neoplasms are a recognized complication of radiation therapy. The majority of benign radiation-induced neoplasms are exostoses (osteochondroma), most commonly occurring in previously normal bone and arising within or at the periphery of the treatment field.[6] Murphy and Blount report cases occurring with doses of 1,600 to 6,425 rads and after latent periods ranging from 9 to 13½ years.[8] These osteochondromas are histologically and radiologically identical to their spontaneously occurring counterparts, although malignant degeneration is less likely than in spontaneous osteochondromata.[6,9] A benign osteoblastoma and an unusual benign cartilaginous tumor have also been reported.[10] These benign radiation-induced neoplasms are more likely in patients treated in early childhood (under 2 years).[11]

The most lethal complication is radiation-induced sarcoma (RIS). In the diagnosis of radiation induced sarcomas, Cahan[12] in 1948, established four criteria: (1) microscopic or radiographic evidence of the nonmalignant nature of the original lesion, (2) malignancy occurring within the radiated field, (3) long latency period—greater than or equal to 5 years between radiation therapy and sarcoma, and (4) histologic proof of sarcoma.

The first criterion has since been modified to include a histologic picture different from the original lesion. This reflects the cases of radiation sarcoma developing in bones irradiated in the treatment of another malignant osseous tumor.[11] With the abandonment of irradiation of benign bone lesions, the majority of RIS patients now have a history of a soft tissue primary with incidental irradiation of underlying bone.[6,13] The histologic and radiographic features of RIS are indistinguishable from spontaneously occurring tumors.[6,13]

Histologically, osteosarcomas are the most common RIS.[12-15] In one study, 66 osteogenic sarcomas (representing approximately 5.5 percent of all osteogenic sarcomas registered between 1921 and 1983 at Memorial Sloan Kettering Cancer Center) occurred in extraosseous or osseous locations as a consequence of therapeutic or incident irradiation.[16] The median latency period between irradiation and development of soft tissue and bone sarcoma was 10.5 years, independent of whether the bone had been normal at the time of irradiation or the radiation had been directed against an osseous lesion. There was a significantly shorter latency period for those 16 years old and under. In this study, the postradiation osteogenic sarcoma was the second most common secondary bone sarcoma, after Paget's sarcoma. The incidence of postradiation osteogenic sarcoma steadily increased with patient age and occurred most commonly in the sixth decade (in comparison with spontaneous lesions, which occur more commonly in the second decade). Additionally, whereas the kneee and distal femur are common sites of spontaneously occurring osteogenic sarcoma, the pelvis, shoulder, upper femur, and flat bones are more commonly involved with postradiation sarcoma.

Fibrosarcoma and chondrosarcoma constitute the second and third most frequent RIS.[11,14] Additionally, there are reports of malignant fibrous histiocytoma (MFH) occurring in irradiated bone.[13,17,18] Vanel et al.[17] reported three cases of bone MFH developing secondary to previous radiation therapy and used CT to demonstrate soft tissue extension of tumor on both sides of a flat bone, distinguishing this from the pattern of localized bone erosion seen with invasion from an adjacent soft tissue tumor.

In a study of 43 patients with RIS of bone secondary to irradiation of soft tissue neoplasms, Smith[13] demonstrated that purely lytic or purely sclerotic patterns were more common than a mixed sclerotic and lytic appearance. He also noted that although the presence of radiation osteitis might assist in establishing a differential diagnosis, it was present in only 50 percent. The presence of pain, a soft tissue mass, and rapid progression of the lesion (without superimposed osteomyelitis) favors sarcoma over radiation osteitis.[6]

Radiation-induced malignancy must also be differentiated from recurring tumor in the irradiated field. Findings of a shorter latency period, a soft tissue mass, and bone erosions or extrinsic invasion favor recurrent tumor. In differentiating radiation-induced malignancy from metastases, the latter usually occur earlier, are not confined to the treatment field, and are usually multiple.[6]

Final diagnosis: Radiation-induced osteogenic sarcoma.

REFERENCES   1. Ewing J: Radiation osteitis. Acta Radiol 6:399, 1926

2. Rubin P, Casarett GW: Growing cartilage and bone. p. 518. In Rubin P, Casarett GW (eds): Clinical Radiation Pathology, Vol. 2. WB Saunders, Philadelphia, 1968

3. Rubin P, Casarett GW: Mature cartilage and bone. p. 557. In Rubin P, Casarett GW (eds): Clinical Radiation Pathology, Vol. 2. WB Saunders, Philadelphia, 1968

4. Bragg DG, Shidnia H, Chu FCH, Higinbotham NL: The clinical and radiographic aspects of radiation osteitis. Radiology 97:103–111, 1970

5. Sengupta S, Prathap K: Radiation necrosis of the humerus: a report of three cases. Acta Radiol 12:313, 1973

6. Dalinka MK, Mazzeo VP, Jr: Complications of radiation therapy. CRC Crit Rev Diagn Imaging 23(3):235, 1985

7. Probert JC, Parker BR: The effects of radiation therapy on bone growth. Radiology 114:155, 1975

8. Murphy FD, Jr. Blount WP: Cartilaginous exostoses following irradiation. J Bone Joint Surg 44:662, 1962

9. Berdon WE, Baker DM, Boyer J: Unusual benign and malignant sequelae to childhood radiation therapy. Am J Roentgenol 93:545, 1965

10. Cohen J, D'Angio GJ: Unusual bone tumors after roentgen therapy of children. Am J Roentgenol 86:502, 1961

11. DeSantos LA, Libshitz HJ: Growing bone and radiation induced neoplasia. p. 151. In Libshitz HI (ed): Diagnostic Roentgenology of Radiotherapy Change. Williams & Wilkins, Baltimore, 1979

12. Cahan WG, Woodard HQ, Higinbotham NL et al: Sarcoma arising in irradiated bone, report of eleven cases. Cancer 1:3, 1948

13. Smith J: Radiation induced sarcoma of bones: clinical and radiographic findings in 43 patients irradiated for soft tissue neoplasms. Clin Radiol 33(2):205, 1982

14. Brady LW: Radiation induced sarcomas of bone. Skel Radiol 4:72, 1979

15. Tefft M, Vawter GF, Mitus A: Second primary neoplasms in children. Am J Roentgenol 103:800, 1968

16. Huvos AG, Woodard HQ, Cahan WG et al: Postradiation osteogenic sarcoma of bone and soft tissues. A clinico pathologic study of 66 patients. Cancer 55(6):1244, 1985

17. Vanel D, Hagay C, Rebibo G et al: Study of three radio-induced malignant fibrous histiocytomas of bone. Skel Radiol 9(3)174, 1983

18. Halpern J, Kopolovic J, Catane R: Malignant fibrous histiocytoma developing in irradiated sacral chordoma. Cancer 53:2661, 1984

Index